Basic Guide to Hospital Public Relations

**American Society
for Hospital Public Relations**
*of the American
Hospital Association*

65910

2nd Edition

American Hospital Publishing, Inc.,
a wholly owned subsidiary of the American Hospital Association

©1984 by American Hospital Publishing, Inc.,
a wholly owned subsidiary
of the American Hospital Association
211 East Chicago Avenue
Chicago, Illinois 60611
Previous edition © 1974,
American Hospital Association

Catalog no. 166121

Tamara Schiller, Editor,
    Book Editorial Department
Marjorie E. Weissman, Manager,
    Book Editorial Department
Dorothy Saxner, Vice-President,
    Book Division

Library of Congress Cataloging in Publication Data
Main entry under title:

A Basic guide to hospital public relations.

    Bibliography: p.
    1. Public relations—Hospitals.   I. American
Hospital Association.   American Society for
Hospital Public Relations.   [DNLM: 1. Hospital
administration.   2. Public relations. WX 150 B261b]
RA965.5.B35   1983   659.2'936211   83-21354
ISBN 0-87258-422-4

Contents

Preface

In the decade since the American Society for Hospital Public Relations (ASHPR) of the American Hospital Association developed its innovative *Basic Guide to Hospital Public Relations,* the concept of public relations in the hospital has matured. Some might say that its role has been superseded by the role of marketing communications, whereas others choose to refer to it by terms other than *public relations.* Nevertheless, goal-oriented, result-oriented communication is more important today for hospitals than it has ever been.

There are many levels of skill and experience in the field of hospital public relations and, in the past decade, public relations has certainly come a long way in terms of both acceptance and sophistication. ASHPR is playing a strong role in this evolution, with programs such as the TOUCHSTONE, which recognizes professionalism in communication programs, and the Professional Achievement Program, which recognizes the qualities of professionalism among members. In addition, regional workshops and an annual educational conference have helped hundreds of hospital public relations practitioners to raise their professional awareness and upgrade the quality of their services to their hospitals and the industry. In this volume, ASHPR again offers useful, practical, proven information to members. As such, the book is geared to those with limited health care or public relations experience who have recently entered the field of hospital public relations.

The first edition of the book was dedicated to "hospital administrators who wish to initiate a public relations program." At present, there are relatively few hospital administrators who have not initiated programs in public relations, recognizing that "PR can pay!" This edition, then, is designed to be a road map for those who accept this notion and who do not wish to fall by the wayside: from the novice public relations director, fresh from school or some other endeavor, to the assistant who has been promoted to the public relations function, to those who are ambitious enough to seek professional advancement in the field of public relations and who want to know the way. It is not an advanced guide, although for the advanced practitioner it might reinforce an idea long held. This book can be used in a self-study or in a regulated program of professional development.

We are in a decade of communication breakthroughs, one of the most exciting and challenging times to consider being a professional communicator. This book is dedicated to those who accept this challenge.

This guide was prepared for the American Society for Hospital Public Relations of the American Hospital Association by Ned B. Barnett, APR, then vice-president, Public Relations, Consumer Affairs, and Marketing, Tennessee Hospital Association, and currently southeastern region marketing manager, Republic Health Corporation, under the auspices of the ASHPR Education Committee. Much appreciation is extended to those who labored over the first edition, which has truly stood the test of time and which was the model and framework on which this new manual was constructed: Wade Edwards, Shirley Bonnem, William J. Brennan, Barbara Traylor, Seymour Leon, Raymond Miller, Joe Sigler, Lillian Sokoll, and Gordon Wright. It is hoped that this effort will be half as durable as theirs has proved to be.

chapter one

Introduction

Health care in America is changing at an almost breakneck pace, and the practice of public relations in the health care setting is changing with it. Public relations is facing an explosion in technology that may, in five years, change not only the face of mass communication media such as television, but also of selective, targeted communication such as public access cable programming and direct computer-to-computer release of news.

Many public relations directors, while thinking themselves insulated in their self-contained hospitals, have unexpectedly become representatives of multimillion-dollar hospital corporations with thousands of employees, facing challenges formerly reserved only for the topflight communicators in the largest firms. Some have adapted, others have not. But none denies that changes are in the works. These changes have introduced new concepts—marketing, positioning, and advertising—to public relations.

However, not every hospital is a multimillion-dollar colossus, and not every hospital communicator is prepared to take on the challenges of such institutions. Yet all communicators need a basic understanding of public relations—and its tools—if they are to compete for public support and understanding in the marketplace of ideas.

Because of its focus, this guide is basic, rather than advanced, and a limited bibliography is included. Hospital public relations, communication, and marketing programs vary according to the hospital's goals, budget, size, and management philosophy. The effectiveness of any program depends upon management's appreciation of the hospital's special communication needs, the establishment of well-defined goals and objectives for the public relations program, and the performance of the person responsible for planning and implementing public relations activities.

Public relations is also a management function in the hospital setting: evaluating public attitudes, identifying policies and procedures of an organization to coincide with public interest or expectation, providing insight as an internal consultant to management, and planning and executing a program of action to earn understanding and acceptance among select publics.

In the past decade, the scope of public relations at various institutions has grown from the traditional house organ and press agentry to a professional communication program that includes the disciplines of advertising, marketing communications, philanthropy, recruiting, and other specific communication-oriented activities. As a result, the specific definition of public relations varies considerably from institution to institution; however, a professional, effective public relations program includes the following:

●Management responsibility reflected on the organizational chart and in the institution's true management team

●Specific goals and objectives that directly support institutional goals and objectives

●Planned and continuous programming aimed at achieving one or more objectives

●Established two-way channels of communication to provide for ongoing evaluation of public attitudes and program effectiveness

●Identification of the institution's policies and procedures from the perspective of the perceived interests of various publics

●Counseling management on the impact that public relations has on the institution's policies and actions

Publicity, including professional internal newsletters and sound media relations based on respect and trust, can and should be elements of a public relations program. However, public relations is far more than publicity. It involves planning, communication, and evaluating programs that promote the goals and objectives of the hospital.

chapter two

The need for public relations

Simply stated, public relations is a systematic program of goal-oriented communication designed to support the needs of the institution. Some professionals have defined it as clear, goal-oriented communication and common sense." In the hospital setting, public relations is a planned program of policies and performance that, if properly communicated, will build confidence and increase understanding and support among selected publics for the institution and its programs or activities.

Perhaps more than ever before, hospitals find themselves compelled to communicate with increasingly skeptical, hostile publics. Consider some current problems: growing criticism of hospital costs, management effectiveness, quality of care and its availability, and the rising specters of state cost regulations and the reaction of the private sector to cost shifting. These problems require careful, continuous public relations and public education programs.

Opinions about hospitals vary according to the sources of information available to different publics, and, within each of those publics, opinions are diversifying. Just as there is no longer a "solid South" in politics, there is no longer a solid physician, community, or employee view of the hospital. Yet never before has there been a greater need for unified, supportive views of the hospital.

Public opinions about a hospital are based first on personal experience with that institution; then on opinions of hospital employees and their families, former patients and their families, others with first-hand information about the hospital, and only then on information derived from the news media or other secondary sources. This primacy of the individual as a source for opinions has a profound implication for hospital public relations practice and highlights the importance of a sound internal relations program as the basis for all external public relations. In addition to providing a firm base for external public relations programs, several other good reasons exist for conducting effective internal relations programs — retention, productivity, and an internal harmony that reflects a pride in the institution.

Externally, public relations serves first as a consultant to management, interpreting society and its expectations to hospital decision makers, ensuring that decisions are not made in an insular vacuum. Beyond that, public relations helps meet institutional goals by developing external support groups that are essential to the long-term survival of the hospital. These groups can assist with development activities, support certificate-of-need applications, encourage high census, and secure a position for the hospital within the community.

Whether or not a hospital has assigned a person — a professional with years of experience or a novice eager to learn and contribute — to public relations responsibilities, the hospital will have communication problems and opportunities that a goal-oriented, well-planned public relations program can solve or exploit, respectively. As hospital management becomes more complicated, requiring more expertise in management fields, the case for public relations professionals on the management team grows stronger. Specialists in public relations can contribute much to the challenges facing hospitals at present and in the future.

*chapter*three

Basic elements of a public relations program

Any hospital public relations program can be organized into eight basic steps.

Establishing goals

The basis of all effective, professional public relations is the setting of department goals and objectives that support existing institutional goals and objectives. Semantically, goals are ideals to strive for, are not subject to measurement, and generally do not change from year to year; objectives are specific and measurable and change as situations change. Both short-term and long-term objectives should be established, and these should be put in writing.

In addition, each program and activity within the overall public relations program should have specific objectives that support specific department goals or objectives and that are in line with institutional goals or objectives. These short-term, project-oriented objectives should be written, but much time should not be spent in polishing the written objective. If the objective cannot be stated in a short paragraph or two, the project probably is not defined or justified adequately and further planning and definition are necessary. With few exceptions, a project should not be undertaken if it does not directly support a department goal or objective. If proposals that do not directly support the overall plan are made frequently, the department or program objectives probably need redefining to include the additional expectations.

Many projects can have both short-term and long-term objectives. In employee recruiting, the long-term objective might be to interest high-school students in health careers, whereas the short-term objective might be to hire new graduates from a local nursing school.

Assessing the current situation

Before a program is developed, an analysis of the external environment, or a situation analysis, must be made. This phase requires a serious evaluation of the need for the program, the target audience, attitudes currently held by that audience, and that audience's receptivity to change through communication. This evaluation can be most effectively done by conducting a professional, scientifically valid survey of the hospital's publics. Although it is true that the results of the situation analysis can have an impact on department and even institutional goals and objectives, the department or program goals and objectives provide a firm footing to conduct the surveys and research that result in the situation analysis.

Gaining access to other surveys

Many surveys are conducted using public funds, with the results entering the public domain. In addition, other demographically sound data, such as census figures, election results, and so forth, can expand greatly the information base from which decisions are made. Another research technique is holding personal discussions with key members of important audience groups, public officials, members of the press, and others whose job it is to understand public attitudes.

Defining problem areas

Using the situation analysis, specific problem areas that require public relations programs must be identified. These areas should become easier to identify when the situation analysis is compared to the hospital's goals and objectives.

The following problems are often found in hospitals, although they and their solutions will vary according to the institution's situation:

● Satisfactorily explaining rising costs and their causes to increasingly skeptical internal and external publics.

- Recruiting employees, especially key groups, such as nurses.
- Attracting volunteers and auxilians to the hospital.
- Defusing press criticism and building a strong, positive relationship with the press based on professionalism and mutual trust.
- Building community and specific public appreciation for the hospital and its programs, including health education, emergency services, obstetrics, and others. This problem often translates into a need to increase the census, using goal-oriented communication techniques aimed at both potential patients and at physicians.
- Developing employee and other internal public support for the institution and raising morale and productivity while combating rumors, inclinations to organize, and so forth.

Identifying pertinent publics

The various publics will naturally divide themselves according to the issues and problem areas defined in the situation analysis. Each situation will have its own set of defined publics. An important concept to remember is that individuals are not irrevocably locked into one category. An employee, for instance, is an internal public for 40 hours per week, but for the other 128 hours that same person may consider himself (and the hospital would be wise to consider him) as a taxpayer, a potential consumer, and as an essentially external public.

The following list includes some typical hospital publics:
- Patients and former patients, classified as inpatient or outpatient
- Employees, classified as full-time or part-time, salaried or hourly, week or weekend, and so forth
- Hospital visitors, perhaps divided into family and friends
- Physicians, divided by specialty and type of privileges
- Government officials
- Auxilians and volunteers
- Trustees
- Hospital donors, divided by personal and corporate givers
- Potential patient populations, such as senior citizens, young children, women of child-bearing age, and so forth
- Hospital suppliers
- Insurance officials
- Students and school guidance counselors
- The media

Targeted communication programs are possible in attempts to reach each of these identified key publics on issues of importance to it and to the hospital. In general, targeted communication efforts are more controllable, more measurable, and more effective than general, mass communication efforts. The only exception to this would be a message that is so universal that all publics should hear it and would be likely to interpret it in the same way. Such messages are few and far between.

Planning the program in detail
An overall public relations program includes a list of problems, applicable objectives, identified publics, and the means of dealing with each problem. The overall program then becomes a list of specific public relations projects, each goal-oriented, measurable, and targeted.

The following outline is an example of an item that might be listed in an overall program. In an actual plan, the lists would be more specific, naming news media and groups, including internal timetables, identifying resources and costs, and so forth.

1. problem
Insufficient number of volunteers to serve actively in the hospital's volunteer program, as defined by the director of volunteer services. (Note: Public relations is a support function; with rare exception, programs begin with a need established by another area of the hospital or by administration. Few programs are conducted to benefit the public relations department itself.)

2. objective
Recruit new volunteers, and return inactive volunteers to service to provide an additional 60 volunteer hours per week within 120 days. (Note: The objective is both measurable and achievable, defining specific targets of performance within a specific timeframe. Open-ended objectives are not measurable and not achievable and, therefore, not really worth doing.)

3. publics involved
Former volunteers, spouses of employees and of the medical staff, members of service organizations, and retired citizens. (For an actual program, this list should be more specific, naming specific groups; for example, Greenville Garden Club, Gray Panthers of Spartanburg, and so forth.)

4. plan
The following activities make up the plan:
●Through interviews with present volunteers, determine factors that motivated participation; through interviews with former volunteers, determine factors that caused them to drop affiliation; through interviews with key or random members of various target publics, identify factors that might motivate future participation.
●Develop support programs that will assist in motivating participation by breaking down barriers identified above, for example, baby-sitting

services for parents and transportation services for elderly volunteers.

● Develop a supporting publicity program that might include feature press coverage on volunteers, public service announcements (PSAs), radio and television talk show appearances, direct mail, and other techniques.

● Develop and implement a plan of public-speaking engagements to target audiences such as garden and women's clubs, senior citizen groups, and PTAs, making use of skilled speakers, supporting audiovisuals, and other resources.

● Evaluate the program to determine whether it meets its objectives. Modify it as appropriate and continue if the need persists.

A formal public relations program must be kept flexible, responsive to changing needs, and oriented to the institution's goals and objectives.

Implementing the public relations program

Having come this far, implementation is almost easy: a detailed road map, that is, a plan that gives destinations, timetable, and budget, is developed in the planning stage.

In a multifaceted program, the most difficult challenge is juggling the many and varied priority projects, making sure that a project or phase of a project has not fallen into the cracks. It is far more important to do a few projects well than it is to do a multitude of projects poorly. A coordinated plan, laid out on a month-by-month calendar and reviewed frequently, can facilitate meeting objectives and help avoid becoming overextended.

Hospitals are administered by professional managers, persons who, by nature and inclination, respect professional management in others. Unfortunately, far too few public relations practitioners have training and specific experience in professional management. The adoption of a professional plan that is goal-oriented and committed to paper can help elevate the management of the program to a level that other professional managers will respect, giving credibility to the program and its manager.

Evaluating the program

Periodic review dates for the overall program, as well as internal review dates for specific projects, should be set. At each review, whether the project is needed, on track, and on budget must be determined. This is why internal measures are necessary for each project and for the program as a whole. Socrates is quoted by Plato as saying, "The life that is unexamined is not worth living." This can be paraphrased for the hospital public relations program: The program that is unmeasured and not evaluated is not worth doing.

chapter four

Responsibilities of the hospital public relations director

The basic scope of a public relations director's responsibility, as defined by the job description, is determined by such factors as the number, size, and significance of various target publics; the attitudes of these publics; the financial resources and size of the hospital; and the commitment from and support provided by the hospital's administration.

The responsibilities of the public relations function can be divided into several broad categories: interpretive and advisory responsibilities, marketing responsibilities, and communication responsibilities. The following activities comprise interpretive and advisory responsibilities:

● Interpret the viewpoints of the hospital's various publics to management and recommend appropriate programs and actions

- Report trends in the attitudes of these publics so that management is prepared to more effectively meet attitudinal changes
- Serve on the hospital's management team, providing the services of in-house public relations counsel and ensuring that public response considerations are evaluated before decisions are made and carried out
- Apprise management of current and contemplated actions and activities of the hospital that will have an impact on the publics' perception of the hospital, and recommend appropriate action
- Gather and analyze data on a continual basis to improve communication systems between the hospital and its publics and to meet the other interpretive and advisory objectives

Marketing responsibilities include the following activities:
- Become intimately familiar with institutional objectives for development of short-term and long-term facilities and services
- In conjunction with institutional planners, develop and conduct market research surveys that will provide support and guidance to the development of institutional plans
- Provide counseling services to planners, helping them to avoid inherent public relations pitfalls and to capitalize on unrecognized advantages and opportunities
- Develop and conduct aggressive, objective-oriented communication programs that are supportive of marketing goals, including census-building, certificate-of-need applications, and franchise consolidation
- Using surveys and other techniques, evaluate marketing and marketing communications programs for their effectiveness

Communication responsibilities of the hospital public relations function are as follows:
- Develop communication materials, such as publications, audiovisuals, media releases, and other tools to promote institutional and departmental goals and objectives
- Target these materials to reach specific publics in a credible fashion with a believable message
- Establish clear, two-way channels of communication between the hospital's various publics and the hospital's management team

Although persons with little training or experience in a hospital or elsewhere cannot be expected initially to perform at the same level as experienced public relations and marketing communications professionals, their goals should include the eventual assumption of the responsibilities and activities of a seasoned professional. Professional organizations, including the Public Relations Society of America, the International Association of Business Communicators, and the American Society of Hospital Public Relations of the American Hospital Association have programs for professional development and accreditation. These groups have chapters nationwide, and they conduct educational programs for communication practitioners throughout the year to aid in developing skills and professionalism.

chapter five

Activities of the
hospital public relations director

Before activities can be undertaken by public relations directors, they must first decide who they are within their organizations — what their roles and their positions are. Many public relations directors have found it effective to adopt the following perspective: Imagine that you are a one-client public relations agency operating outside of the organization, yet dependent upon its success for your own. By viewing yourself as an outsider, you can maintain an objective perspective that will become an important asset. In addition, with but a single client, it is imperative to keep that client happy by doing your professional best at all times. By adopting this perspective, directors of public relations enhance their professionalism and productivity, even before the first step toward serving the institution is taken.

The major public relations responsibilities of interpreting and advising, marketing, and communicating are met by performing principal activities that are presented below. These activities are described as undertaken by an experienced public relations director. Again, all new public relations directors (regardless of title, and there are many titles in circulation) should personally aspire to undertake these activities as they gain experience and knowledge.

Research

Determining attitudes and opinions of various publics; identifying problem areas, opportunities, and possible solutions; and interpreting this information for management are important first steps in the public relations function. To be fully informed on present and contemplated objectives of the hospital, hence, to be able to design appropriate research studies and programs, the public relations director should serve on the hospital management team and attend meetings of the hospital governing board. Virtually no meeting or piece of information should be denied the public relations director. As a result, only a person of the highest personal integrity can succeed in this demanding position; personal discretion has never been more important than in the present competitive environment.

Planning

Planning is essential to the success of any public relations program. A basic public relations plan that establishes specific objectives, activities, timing, budgeting, and other factors can be a tool, rather than a chore. A sound plan is a document that management will understand, and it will give management a basis for evaluating the performance of the public relations department. A carefully thought-out plan can assist the public relations director to cover all the bases and to avoid inadvertantly overlooking important hospital priorities in the rush of day-to-day activities.

An effective plan is goal-oriented and measurable. It includes review and revision activities that will keep the plan relevant and on target.

Coordination

Each department or subgroup of the hospital has the tendency to want to communicate its message in its own way. This practice can result in a confused cacophony that makes little sense from the varied perspectives of the hospital's publics and adds nothing to a positive impression of the hospital as an institution. Advising and counseling other department managers about how activities of their departments involve public relations; making available technical skills of public relations staff for communication programs of other departments; and gently working behind the scenes with tact and good will to enforce the necessity of a coordinated message are all activities called for in effective public relations managers. It is not an easy job; it is especially vital, however, in a competitive environment.

Counseling

Counseling management on the public relations implications of policies, plans, and practices in the hospital is a vital role, calling for personal credibility that can grow only through a good performance proven over time. However, hospitals should never make decisions without considering their impact on their publics. In fact, this is one of the prime justifications for the public relations function serving at the management level.

On occasion, the public relations department will be called upon to provide assistance to other departments and others in the hospital community, assistance that at first seems beyond its usual scope. As long as cooperation does not seriously impede the completion of priority projects, being a team player and pitching in is best. This attitude of cooperation will bring dividends of cooperation in the future.

Marketing

Marketing and marketing communications are becoming increasingly important roles for professional public relations directors. Marketing communications makes use of all available communication tools: advertising, public relations (traditional tools such as publications and brochures, press releases, broadcast exposure, and public meetings), and others. Marketing pulls together the activities of research, planning, advising, and coordinating and combines them with effective, goal-oriented communication designed to assist the hospital's development of its franchise within the community—that base of support and service that justifies the institution's very existence.

Fund raising

The raising of funds to support the hospital and its programs through charitable giving and related means, whether assigned the term *fund raising, development,* or *philanthropy,* operates hand in glove with marketing and public relations functions in some hospitals. Although development activities are often carried out one-on-one by staff assigned solely to this purpose or by willing community volunteers, successful development programs are supported effectively by a strong public relations communication program that is in line with the marketing plans of the hospital. There is a real danger in a hospital development program that conducts communication that is out of sync with other hospital communication programs. Such a conflict can injure the entire hospital communication effort and the programs the effort was designed to support. As a result, the public relations director should be intimately involved in the communication function of the development program.

Recruitment
If recruitment of additional hospital and medical staff is an institutional priority, communication must be designed to promote and enhance this function for all departments and programs in the hospital. Public relations must be intimately involved in these communication activities, as successful recruitment of qualified staff or physicians is frequently essential to the success of marketing plans. Through its coordination efforts, public relations can facilitate this success.

Media relations
Media relations is one of the obvious and traditional roles of hospital public relations. A premature "leak" of information about a hospital's plans for expansion; the unauthorized release of patient information that violates a patient's privacy; or the expression of a view contrary to the hospital's position by someone speaking "for the hospital" can injure the hospital's reputation for accuracy, honesty, and professionalism, and may cause immeasurable damage by weakening the hospital's market position or landing the hospital in court with an invasion of privacy suit. Just as public relations directors should never take an active role in the delivery of patient care, those in other areas of the hospital should not communicate with the press, except in cooperation with the public relations director.

Media relations activities include developing institutionwide policies for the release of information to the press and the public; planning, creating, and placing publicity material with the appropriate news outlets; assisting reporters in obtaining accurate information from appropriate hospital representatives; and other activities designed to promote positive, professional press relations.

Public relations staff should always strive to be open and honest with the press; one misleading statement can destroy individual credibility and the credibility of the hospital, making the job difficult or, perhaps, impossible.

Production of materials
As an effective medium for patient education, community relations, and a host of other communication

needs, audiovisuals are vitally important to public relations directors and their programs. Some hospitals have no audiovisual capabilities, permitting public relations directors to create their own programs to suit the hospitals' specific needs. Other hospitals have audiovisual capabilities operated by an education or personnel department. Cooperation with these areas is far more cost-effective than setting up a competing department; however, conflicting priorities may be difficult to overcome, as may the problem of inconsistent messages being produced and disseminated. The hospital public relations department is charged with primary responsibility for the maintenance of the hospital's image to various publics. Unless public relations has some measure of responsibility for audiovisual communication production, the hospital may find itself producing communication tools that are at variance with or even at cross-purposes to the communication goals of the institution itself. Useful audiovisual tools for the communication program include slide-taped presentations, videotapes, and audiotapes. The use of the latter two with the news media is a new and growing area in public relations.

The development, production, and extensive distribution of hospital publications, such as newsletters for internal and external consumption, annual reports, booklets, brochures, and flyers, seem to be some of the most securely rooted functions of the public relations department. In creating publications, bear in mind that an increasing number of persons cannot read or read so poorly that they choose not to read. This factor can have profound implications for both patient and employee communication. In an attempt to overcome this difficulty (and for other good reasons), some hospitals are producing videotaped "patient brochures" that are shown over closed-circuit television and video "employee newsletters," (see appendix C). However, for many audiences and for many purposes, publications are the communication tools of choice and should remain so for some time to come.

Special events

The planning and execution of special events are often delegated to the public relations department. In some cases, these programs are also incorporated into the overall public relations program and are aimed at building good will or generating support for a certificate-of-need application or another hospital goal. Special events can be geared to internal publics, external publics, or a mix. Such events may include tours, anniversary celebrations, National Hospital Week (sponsored by the American Hospital Association), community education programs, and a host of others. Lists of special health-related days, weeks, and months are published annually by ASHPR. These can help with planning programs, allowing a hospital to take advantage of activities that, presumably, are already receiving public attention, such as heart month (February) or hypertension month (May). There is even a public relations week!

Speaker's bureau

A hospital speaker's bureau, managed by the hospital's public relations division and consisting of speakers such as trustees, administrators, managers, and perhaps physicians, can facilitate putting skilled experts in a position to tell all or a part of the hospital's story. Various forums for speaker's bureau presentations include civic groups, talk shows, and others. In addition to arranging and coordinating the speaking engagements, the public relations division has two important roles: training potential speakers to put their own and the hospital's best foot forward and preparing speech texts, audiovisuals, and handouts to make the presentation a success. Naturally, publicity for the events should also be developed, as appropriate.

Administration

As a department, public relations must be managed as any other. This involves personnel and budget in addition to program management, roles that too many otherwise professional public relations directors find difficult. There are many useful texts on departmental management that can be applied to public relations, as well as other departments; furthermore, organizations such as American Society for Hospital Public Relations, Public Relations Society of America, and International Association of Business Communications conduct periodic workshops on program management that can be helpful in sorting through the maze of challenges in budgeting and personnel management.

Community involvement

Many hospitals encourage or even require management-level personnel to participate in community groups such as Rotary, Civitan, Lions, or other groups. Such encouragement can benefit the public relations program in two ways. First, by participating personally, the public relations director has the opportunity to meet community leaders in a forum away from the hospital, to continually assess attitudes about the hospital. Second, the public relations department can work with other involved department managers to gain access to important community groups for speaker's bureau presentations and similar efforts.

Education

Hospital public relations directors should strive to learn all they can about the hospital industry, as well as about hospital and department management and financing, to do their jobs effectively. But more important, in the competitive market environment that hospitals are facing, continuing professional education in public relations has become essential.

In addition, public relations as a discipline is changing rapidly; in fact, some professionals estimate that the half-life of a professional public relations education is just five years. Therefore, education is a constant challenge to and a constant opportunity for the public relations professional.

Evaluation

The public relations program must be evaluated periodically, first, to see if it has been meeting its goals and objectives and, second, to see if those goals and objectives are still in line with institutional goals and objectives. A periodic self-evaluation should be conducted by the public relations director. Using the written public relations plan as a benchmark, he should look carefully at the program: Have the objectives been met? Is the program within budget? Are ongoing programs on schedule? Does the plan itself actually serve institutional goals and objectives?

Periodically, perhaps on a quarterly basis, the supervisor who oversees the public relations department (ideally the hospital CEO) should also evaluate the public relations program, using the same criteria as the self-evaluation. In this way, the public relations director will have the opportunity to modify the planned activities to meet the changing needs and expectations of the institution.

The specific activities of a public relations director will depend on the local hospital situation, the person's individual and staff skills, the resources available to support public relations, and the publics involved. Tailoring public relations programs for different publics is an essential activity, and subsequent sections of this manual will describe program possibilities aimed at a variety of specific publics.

Selection and use of consultants

As a part of the evaluation procedure, an outside perspective may prove useful. In this case, a public relations consultant may be called in. Consultants can be found to fill almost any conceivable need. The communication field is particularly well-stocked with skilled consultants who offer value received for their services. Unfortunately, the field also has its share of self-proclaimed experts who will take the hospital's money but offer little of value in return. By approaching the field of consultants carefully, the problems connected with the selection of the person best suited to meet the hospital's needs can be avoided.

Identifying needs With what do you need help? A complete audit of the communication program? A marketing survey? The development of a slide presentation? A clear needs statement will assist in the selection process.

Identifying the budget How much can the hospital afford to spend in time and money to secure the right consultant and conduct the project at hand? Cost will also help select the appropriate consultant.

Selecting the consultant Contacting colleagues, professional organizations, and state hospital associations for recommendations will turn up some good leads. From several candidates, a consultant who seems to be most competent within the budgetary restrictions can be selected. Checking references is a must.

Defining expectations A letter of agreement or a contract should state specifically what is expected from the consultant and what and when the hospital will pay for those services. This will avoid misunderstand-ings and disappointments later. If deadlines are important, they should be specified in the agreement.

Laying the groundwork Before consultants come on site, they should be provided with all pertinent background information. This will ensure that the hospital gets the most value for the time spent working with the consultant.

Planning ahead After determining what the consultant intends to do while on site, a schedule of activities, meetings, conferences, and work sessions should be prepared. This planning will avoid wasted time and facilitate meeting the consulting objectives.

Acting on the consultant's report Far too often, consultants' reports are considered the final step in solving the problem. Having invested time and money in a consultant, the best use of that investment is to act. Putting the findings to work or using the product or tool the consultant has produced is a must to solve any problems or bring about change.

Evaluating the process An evaluation that measures the success and applicability of the consultant's end product and critiques the entire process will assist in future selection and use of consultants. This necessary final step should not be forgotten.

*chapter*six

Employee relations

To avoid confusing and wasteful duplication of effort and to ensure that all communication is goal-oriented, all public relations activities should be coordinated through one individual — the public relations director. However, public relations is everybody's business. All hospital employees should be aware of and continually reminded that the hospital is judged every day by their actions and appearance and that this judgment can affect their jobs and their lives.

Effective hospital public relations begins with employees, their attitudes, and the quality of services they provide. If your house is in order, you will have a good foundation for launching your public relations program and achieving your departmental and institutional goals. Positive employee relations should be the product of carefully planned, well-executed programs, rather than the result of the daily ups and downs that everyone experiences. Certainly, positive employee relations begin with person-oriented working conditions, an attractive environment, caring supervision, and adequate pay scales. However, there are several other factors, public relations factors, that can reinforce positive employee relations, leading directly to improved morale, retention, productivity, and a positive image among external publics. These factors are discussed below.

Orientation

It is vital to the well-being of the hospital's patients that all employees know their hospital, its policies, procedures, and expectations. Orientation for new employees and periodic reorientation for other employees is usually the combined responsibility of the personnel department, the public relations department, and the department in which the employee works. A well-informed, supportive employee is better equipped to be an effective representative of the hospital. To give employees a concept of the role they play in the overall operation of the hospital, orientation should cover the following:

● Organization, including ownership, financing, supervision, governance, and regulatory restrictions
● Ethics of patient and employee relationships
● Emphasis on empathy with the patient as a person, stressing that health care is a *service* industry and that it is on service that the hospital will be judged
● A tour or audiovisual preview of all departments and areas of the hospital
● Safety and disaster preparedness
● The role of auxiliary and volunteer services (New volunteers can also go through this orientation program.)
● The factors behind hospital costs
● Personal health and hygiene
● The importance of effective hospital public relations, including the direct and indirect benefits to employees and employees' role in creating and maintaining effective public relations, on the job and off
● Common sense and courtesy tips for contact with patients and visitors
● Use of internal hospital communication, with stress on the importance of employee feedback
● The role of the hospital in the community in addition to providing treatment: the economic impact of the hospital, the resources it provides beyond inpatient care, and so forth
● Personnel services available to employees, including credit unions, health service benefits, and so forth
● Personnel policies and benefits
● Grievance procedure or other appropriate channels available to employees who have an employment-related problem

Orientation programs may be presented in group assemblies of new employees or in individual briefings by hospital department heads using a prepared outline of subjects to be covered. In either event, the assimilation of employees is far too important a task to be overlooked or delegated to untrained, ill-prepared personnel.

Information and communication

Employees have a strong need to know what is happening at their place of employment. Security is a very basic psychological need and motivator, and a lack of information quickly equates to a lack of security. Morale suffers, and employees start looking for working environments in which they feel safer. In addition, knowing what's happening at the institution before it is in the newspaper allows employees to take pride in being informed about their institution.

The tools and techniques for disseminating information to employees vary widely with circumstances. Small hospitals may use a central bulletin board, whereas large hospitals may have a printed daily bulletin or newsletter. Techniques that have proved effective are:

● Employee meetings, including open forums that feature give-and-take between employees and administrators. (This requires a very secure administrator to be effective.)

● Bulletin boards with regular postings, such as immediately following board or management meetings
● Slide shows, videotapes, or other audiovisuals that can be transported from work station to work station or put on in-house closed-circuit television
● Brochures and other printed employee information
● Newsletters of varying frequency, from quarterly magazines to daily bulletins
● Direct mail of flyers, which has the added advantage of reaching the family, as well as employees

Disseminating information should not be confused with communication, which is two-way in nature. However, it should not be downgraded just because it is all channeled in one direction; it is important in maintaining good employee relations.

Public relations programs that not only provide opinion, but also invite feedback are essential to effective employee relations, and these programs reflect a communication rather than an information orientation. Most of the techniques and tools described for information can be applied here, as long as a feedback mechanism is provided. A column for letters in the newsletter and a suggestion box are traditional methods for inviting feedback. Using audiovisual news reports and open forums to solicit feedback are new approaches. Any approach that works is worth exploring because of the essential nature of feedback to effective public relations.

Learning opportunities

In addition to continuing education in the hospital and outside seminars or workshops, hospitals can plan monthly sessions featuring speakers and discussions on investments, personal financial management, job attitudes, income tax returns, insurance, upcoming elections, and other topics of interest to employees. Other programs of this nature can include wellness programs to help employees stop smoking, lose weight, get into shape, or cope with stress. These programs demonstrate to the employee and to others that the hospital's commitment to wellness goes beyond its treatment of patients.

Social activities

Many hospitals sponsor annual or periodic social events for employees and their families, such as picnics, Christmas and other seasonal parties, block seating at athletic events, bowling and softball teams, open houses, and a host of others. The key to effective social events is that they make the hospital fun, at least for a little while, and that they give the employees status and position that have little or nothing to do with the jobs they do at the hospital.

Combating rumors

In any organization, rumors are spread before management can offer adequate explanation, assuming management has the internal credibility to offer such explanation. Some hospitals have found a rumor box system successful. The box is placed in a well-trafficked spot, and employees are invited to jot down any rumors they hear and to drop the information in the box. The box should be checked regularly, the rumor investigated, and a response to that rumor posted on the bulletin board next to the box. Another technique involves the use of a telephone-answering machine that permits employees to anonymously phone in rumors they hear. A mechanism to respond to rumors should be established along with this technique. However, the most effective check on rumors is a vigorous, proactive communication program that gets the facts out before the rumors can begin. The best way to prevent rumors is to tell employees the truth, which is why so many hospitals have developed mechanisms to quickly and accurately summarize board decisions and management plans.

Technology and tools

Technological breakthroughs offer new opportunities to communicate with employees, though many traditional approaches continue to have value. Interactive telephone systems now permit hospitals to record daily news for employees on an in-house telephone line, then invite comment and response. In addition to saving paper and printing costs, this cuts the time needed to get the word out. The same technology can be used to give patients a daily summary of world, national, local, and hospital news, a welcome service for shut-ins.

Closed circuit television can provide an added dimension to in-house communication. With even modest production facilities, a hospital can put together a daily news summary that can be broadcast, on a regular schedule, to patient rooms and employee common areas. Television is a very credible medium and can enhance a message's inherent believability. However, hospitals without this capability can still post a daily news bulletin to maintain a flow of information at a low cost.

Less immediate communication can be accomplished through the publication of periodic newsletters or magazines distributed at work stations or mailed to homes. In addition, video or audiovisual news programming featuring the hospital and staff can be distributed for viewing at work stations during breaks.

Budgets can be the restraining factors in some of the more advanced techniques, but often existing technology can be put to work for the hospital's in-house communication efforts. For example, a hospital with an in-house computer system might put a daily news summary in the computer, permitting individuals to call it up at their work station. Print-outs could be made for those persons without terminals. Computers have an immediacy and a perceived infallibility that can be used for public relations work in some situations.

chapter seven

Other internal relations

Employees are not the only internal groups in hospitals that demand the attention of public relations. Most internal groups need special, tailored programs to meet their specific information and communication needs. The demands on public relations from these groups will vary widely with the institution.

Governing board

Members of the hospital governing board comprise a very special public, one that must be dealt with carefully and effectively. As with volunteers, these individuals maintain an important link between the hospital and the community. Though they are called on to make decisions that can have a drastic impact on the future of the hospital, they are not always fully informed on health care issues.

Hospital board relations must be conducted under the specific direction and guidance of the hospital's administrator. Hospital chief executive officers are generally hired by hospital boards to operate the hospitals under their guidance, whereas all other hospital employees are hired, directly or indirectly, by the chief executive officers to help them carry out their mandate from the board. For this reason, if no other, all board relations must be carried out under the administrator's direction. Even in hospitals owned by multihospital systems, the chief executive officer is the key link to the board.

Board relations can begin with orientation of new board members, an orientation that should go far beyond the buildings and services of the hospital and extend to the issues facing the hospital and the health care industry. From this base, board relations can include gathering periodic abstracts of important articles on health care issues (public relations directors should be reading these, anyway). Some hospitals send, for information purposes, copies of press releases to board members at the time they are distributed to the press, then send clippings of important local press coverage. These can serve as a window for the board members, showing them how the public, through the press, views hospitals. One other notion: Board members are, at some hospitals, called on to answer questions from the press or to function under the full glare of press coverage. A course in dealing with the media, either a high-cost profes-

sional course or an in-house effort conducted by the public relations department, can help ease their minds in this area and can improve press coverage, as well.

Physicians

Members of the medical staff can be considered either as internal or external. Either way, they form a vital public for the hospital, a public that can make or break the institution. Constantly staying one step ahead of their needs and expectations is a difficult, but important, role for the hospital public relations program.

As with employees, physicians like to be informed and consulted on plans and projects that will affect them. Medical staff meetings, a medical staff newsletter, and other avenues of communication provide important links between the institution and the physicians, if used properly.

Volunteers and auxilians

These dedicated persons provide an important link between the hospital and the community, yet too often they are ignored as a public to be reached through effective communication. Their support may, in fact, be less oriented toward the hospital than to the patient. A significant number of volunteers actively resent their hospitals for failing to show proper appreciation for their efforts, yet they continue from a dedication or commitment to the patient.

Volunteer relations begins with improving their image with hospital employees. Employees should know what volunteers have been doing and the value of their activities to the hospital, patients, and employees. The second stage of such a program focuses on communicating with the volunteers themselves, helping them feel like insiders at the hospital. This stage includes keeping them abreast of hospital activities and aspirations and finding out what interests and concerns they, as volunteers, share. The final stage might be promoting volunteer activities to external publics, both to give further recognition to this group and to help with future recruiting.

Patients

Patients are a captive but fleeting public, truly representing a cross-section of society. The care they receive will form the greatest part of their impression of the hospital (hence, the need for effective employee relations). Therefore, specific programs have been developed to meet the needs of patients and the hospital.

Patient admission brochures are a tradition with hospitals. However, many patients either cannot read well enough to appreciate them or have too little interest or energy to make the effort. As a result, many progressive hospitals are moving to a closed-circuit admissions videotape or some other audiovisual program that will orient the patient to the hospital. This can pave the way for video patient education, an important service.

Visitors

Closely allied with the patient is the visitor. The same restrictions about reading skills and interest can apply here, but opportunities for videotaped communication may be limited to patient waiting areas. One hospital chose to connect the television in the emergency waiting area to an in-house channel that broadcast nothing but health education and hospital orientation programming. A few visitors complained about missing soap operas or football, but most appreciated the information.

Problem solving through communication

The best way to handle any problem is to avoid it. The next best way is to handle it immediately — before it has a chance to fester. This is especially true when dealing with the human element.

A hot line can provide a low-cost, low-risk path to improved two-way communication. As such, it can be a most effective management tool, as well as a communication tool. Opened to patients and visitors, it can help to identify patient problems while that patient is still in the hospital, when the problem can still be resolved. Opened to the employees, it can head off unrest, improve job satisfaction, and give the administration an "open" image. Opened to the public, the physicians, the board, and others, it can be an important new source of information—and information is vital to the successful operation of a hospital in a complex environment.

The basic tool is a telephone, in house or out of house, depending on the target audience, which may include all employees, patients, even the community, and a recorder for the phone. Here is how it works:

Step 1—commitment Hospital administrators must be firmly committed to the program. Their authority and support will make the program. They should be the voice of the recordings, the person behind seeking solutions to the problems.

Step 2—promotion The target audiences must understand both the mechanics of the system and its purpose. Their understanding and support will help make the hot line a success. Once the system has been promoted to employees, a coordinated campaign to reach other audiences—patients and visitors—should be developed.

Written communication can include admission packets, "point-of-purchase" tent cards for bedside tables, visitors' brochures, even patient newslettters. Nonwritten backup systems are important for those who will not take the time to read. In-house closed-circuit television can be one medium: A commercial for the hot line can explain its purpose. Volunteers, chaplains, other support personnel, and the patient care staff can discuss it, promote it, and explain it. (This is why promotion must begin with employees.)

Finally, a dedicated direct telephone line—a red hot-line telephone—properly indicated with signs or handouts, can be put in the visitors' waiting area.

Step 3—operations To be effective, all complaints must be quickly checked out. Responses must be made to the complainant promptly, generally within 24 to 48 hours. Once the hot line has a reputation for working, it will work.

Many times, the complainant just needs an outlet, a bit of interest, a sounding board. Providing that outlet, that chance to voice a complaint, may, in effect, nip the problem in the bud. And in those cases when more is required, at least the problem will be identified and can be handled.

However, a hot line is just one tool, serving a limited, but important, purpose in the realm of patient communication. This too-often overlooked area can be approached from a number of different vantages. Far too many hospitals settle for the admitting packet or brochure and think they have done a good job. In reality, they haven't scratched the surface.

A daily or weekly newsletter can be mimeographed or photocopied at low cost. Contents should include news of activities at the hospital that day or week; a few select facts about the hospital yesterday, today, and tomorrow; and local news excerpted or summarized from the daily paper. Patients sometimes feel cut off, and they want to know what is going on. To reduce the effort required for a daily newsletter to an effective minimum, items from the newspaper or from the latest employee newsletter can be pasted together and quickly printed for the patients. Distribution can be done by dietary with lunch, or by volunteers on their daily rounds.

Another tool is the phone-in. A 90-second to 5-minute daily message using a telephone playback unit can cover events at the hospital; provide a brief, interesting message about the hospital; or list key items from the morning paper. This system has to be continually promoted to reach the changing patient population, but it costs little. An added advantage is that all patients, regardless of literacy levels, can use this system.

For hospitals with in-house closed-circuit television systems that broadcast health education and health care programming to patients, a noon news program can be fun and effective.

Using a simple set, a short program of news that includes events at the hospital, items from the daily paper, and plugs for the hospital can be put together. Properly promoted, this tool can increase the viewership of the in-house system, as well as reach patients. The TV system will become more visible and, therefore, more effective.

A wholly unnecessary problem area comes from patients' lack of awareness of services they receive. For example, a woman complained in a postdischarge survey that her room had not been cleaned for four straight days. Research quickly established that she had been in physical therapy while her room was cleaned. The solution was to leave tent cards in rooms that are cleaned when the patient is out. The card has information about where to complain if the clean-up is not successful.

This system of brief, ongoing communication with patients, advising them of services received, can leave the patient with a positive image of the hospital.

chapter eight

News media relations

Effective news media relations are based on credibility, professionalism, and mutual trust. These are not created overnight. The hospital must appreciate and respect the role of the press to disseminate news of interest to readers, viewers, or listeners, and the reporters and editors must appreciate the hospital's overriding commitment to protecting the rights and privacy of its patients.

The past three decades have seen the breakdown of the concept of mass media into a series of targeted media that can deliver specific audiences for specific purposes. Radio networks in the pre-television days and the mass magazines such as *Look, Life,* and *The Saturday Evening Post* in the early days of television provided communicators with true mass media outlets. At present, these media have become segmented, while television has assumed the mantle of the "mass medium." However, in the early 1980s this concept is already disintegrating as cable, satellite, local access, videotape, disk, and other uses for television are breaking down the mass audience. In 1978, John Chancellor, NBC anchor, predicted to the national convention of the PRSA that within 10 years television networks would cease to exist as presently constituted. In the interim, Cable News Network has arisen to justify Chancellor's opinion that only news programming would survive as a national "net," while ABC, CBS, and others have entered the cable and packaged communication markets to supplement and, some believe, eventually replace the current mass market network entertainment formats.

These moves, when coupled with the deregulation of broadcasting that has lifted much of the public service requirement, have a profound impact on the practice of public relations. There is no consensus on the future of public relations in a totally segmented communication system. However, it is clear that segmentation provides the opportunity to direct specific messages to specific audiences, as opposed to general messages to general audiences. To those who can master the new opportunities being presented, this holds a clear advantage in tightly controlled, goal-oriented communication.

Strategy of communication

Press relations is a given in most public relations operations. It is one of the unquestioned roles of the public relations division. Perhaps it is time to question this.

All of the hospital's communication efforts should be goal-oriented, and communication through and with the press should be no different. Before that news release is sent out or that reporter's question answered, the following questions should be asked:
- Why release this information?
- What do I hope to accomplish?
- Who should receive this information?
- What hospital goals will be advanced by this release?
- What will happen if I don't release this information?

Another question logically develops from the above list: What is news? The following events and activities are possible news or feature material to send to broadcasters or newspapers:
- New equipment
- Board appointments and elections
- Department head and staff appointments
- Auxiliary-sponsored activities
- National Hospital Week
- Hospital speaker's bureau engagement announcements

- New high-technology services
- Hospital personnel receiving awards or recognition
- Financial information about the hospital
- Case studies reflecting advanced medical care
- Holiday activities at the hospital
- Service and rate changes
- Unusual hobbies or activities of employees
- Hospital service anniversaries (personnel and facilities)
- "Day in the life" of employees or volunteers
- Community education announcements

In other words, communication efforts must serve some established department or hospital goal. Of course, it almost never pays to be uncooperative with members of the press, and any decision to avoid answering a question must be carefully considered for short-term and long-term consequences.

Dealing with the media
Hospitals should develop and attempt to enforce an official policy for working with the press. This may be based on one of the many press codes that have been developed by the American Hospital Association or by state and local hospital associations and councils. State laws vary with respect to what patient information must be released; beyond such requirements, hospitals enter the shaky area of potentially violating a patient's right to privacy. A clear, easily comprehended release or waiver incorporated into the admission form offers a measure of protection; however, court cases can be avoided if one errs on the side of protecting the patient. This, of course, can complicate press relations.

Copies of hospitals' written press policies should be available to all hospital employees. Special emphasis should be given to those employees who may be called on to make a statement to the press when the public relations office is closed, as is often the case when accident victims are admitted at night. If night supervisors or others who may receive press calls know the press policies, they can prevent a lawsuit or, at least, embarrassment.

Although it is important to know the audience, the capabilities, the deadlines, the restrictions, and the policies of each medium and news media outlet, there are certain basic guidelines that can be used in dealing with all reporters and editors:
- Be honest. Being untruthful or half-truthful to make the hospital look good will destroy the press's confidence in the hospital and its public relations director. This does not require that public relations staff seek out opportunities to disclose the negative side of its hospital's operations; it does oblige it to avoid cover-ups.

●Be accurate. All names, times, and statements should be checked before releasing information. All nonroutine releases should be approved by the chief executive officer to be sure the information is correct and conforms with policy.

●Be concise and professional. Competition for space in newspapers and time on the air is fierce. Copy stands a better chance of being used if it is prepared in good journalistic style and format. However, it is often trimmed, rewritten, or not used at all. This is to be expected. *Public relations directors should never question an editor for cutting or discarding their releases or features.*

●Be appreciative. For a particularly good play of a story, a thank-you call or a note to the reporter or editor is in order. There is an art to saying thanks, which should be cultivated. For broadcasters, a letter to the Federal Communications Commission's license renewal file on behalf of the station is a very valuable way of saying thank you to a reporter or news director. A copy should be sent to the station manager. In print, a thank-you letter to the publisher or senior editor might be more appropriate. Whatever the method, the thanks should be specific.

Code of cooperation

The administrator or public relations director for the hospital should be the one person who reporters and media representatives know to contact when they have questions. Hospital staff members should be directed to channel all media inquiries through this designated person, except in limited, clearly defined areas such as condition reports. This rule can be difficult to enforce, but it can greatly simplify the public relations-media relations process.

Recognizing the valuable function of newspapers, radio, and television and being aware that the first obligation of physicians and hospitals is to safeguard the life, health, and legal rights — including privacy — of the patients, hospitals are urged to adopt a media guide or code of cooperation that defines which information related to patients can be released and which must be embargoed. As laws vary from state to state, state hospital associations and hospital attorneys should be consulted in drafting this code. Many hospitals choose to incorporate this code into their published policies.

If possible, the code of cooperation should be jointly developed and formally adopted by hospitals and representatives of the local media. If not, the code should be shared with the local news media. In any case, when certain information cannot be released, an explanation should be provided. To give the press a terse "no comment" will guarantee deteriorating press relations and negative coverage, as reporters seek to find what you are "trying to hide."

Journalistic skills

In dealing with the press, an understanding of its workings seems desirable. In past years, this equated to seeking public relations directors from the ranks of former journalists; this is still a common practice. However, an increasing number of public relations directors come from the ranks of public relations (which often includes reportorial training), marketing, English (which seldom includes reportorial training), or a related field.

Public relations practitioners will benefit from enrolling in a correspondence course, evening program, or short-term college program to receive an introduction to newsgathering and reporting. Courses such as Introduction to Journalism may be historical rather than experiential and may not be what is needed. However, introductory courses in broadcast news have value, especially for those practicing public relations in the major market areas. If good programs are not available, contact local reporters and editors to learn more about how they do their jobs.

Training in public relations teaches the graduate to work effectively, in a goal-oriented fashion, with a variety of reporters and editors. This is highly recommended for those with a journalistic background who want to master the intricacies of public relations.

In press relations, editors and reporters set a high premium on accuracy and style. A basic journalism text, a good dictionary, and a press stylebook (available from AP, UPI, or the *New York Times*) are as useful as a thesaurus to the public relations writer.

Some public relations directors give Christmas presents to reporters to show appreciation. This is neither necessary nor appropriate and can result in hard feelings by those who may be left out. Many reporters refuse or are forbidden to accept such gifts. However, a press recognition program that gives reporters and editors solid evidence of the hospital's appreciation, in the form of a certificate or plaque, can be very valuable. The key to appreciation, however, is sincerity.

Press coverage

Before press coverage is solicited, the goal of obtaining the coverage should be understood, and the impact of negative press coverage carefully evaluated. Once secure in the knowledge that being prepared can engender, the press can be invited to the hospital. Many think that this means a press conference and, perhaps, it does. However, a press conference is the most potentially volatile, dangerous forum for meeting the press. One should be conducted only if there is solid news of widespread interest and if a press conference is the only way of informing the press and the community of the news. The following problems can easily crop up during a press conference:

● No one attends, or only a few reporters attend
● More reporters attend than can be handled
● Questioning strays from the topic to areas the person presiding is not prepared to discuss
● The person presiding at the conference gets flustered or angry at the questions

Therefore, satisfactory solutions to all of these possibilities must be prepared before a press conference is called.

Representatives of the press may be invited to cover significant events or activities at the hospital. Invitations can be made by telephone or letter. If the meeting is a luncheon or dinner, the press should be invited to join in the meal. Some will accept, some cannot. Additional preparations to handle the press are necessary, such as having handouts available, making room for television cameras, and being on hand to answer questions. Television coverage requires interesting visuals and a short "sound bite" — an audio "actuality" that adds realism and immediacy to the coverage; radio has similar sound requirements, using actualities perhaps as short as 10 seconds. Newspaper reporters like background facts, attributable quotes, photos of participants, and material that can quickly be translated into charts, graphs, or maps, as appropriate. By catering to the needs of the specific media involved, the chances of favorable coverage are increased significantly.

Reporters and editors

Most hospital news will be handled by the city desk of daily newspapers covering a hospital's service area, but some have not only reporters assigned to the hospital beat but also science and medical reporters to handle scientific news and features. Public relations directors should know their city editors and specialized reporters and channel their stories to the proper person: auxiliary functions and receptions to the society or life-style editor, research stories to the science reporter, financial stories to the business editor, and so forth.

Weeklies usually do not have such large staffs, and the contact person is generally the editor or general assignments reporter. If hospital news is consistently assigned to one reporter, it is safe to contact that reporter directly.

Deadlines

Media deadlines, be they for daily papers, weeklies, or broadcasters, must be learned and respected for timely release of news. There are no standards for deadlines as existed in the past. New technology has permitted newspapers to "go to bed" just minutes before the presses role, and many television stations have gone to a live interview format within the news program. Local news outlets can provide information on deadlines, but the public relations staff must be sensitive to changes.

When reporters and editors are on deadline, they have no time for anything but the hottest breaking news. The courtesy and consideration of not disturbing them with relatively minor items at these times will be repaid.

However, a reporter's deadlines are not yours. If reporters call right before deadline (and they will), they will pressure for a quick answer. Be sure the facts are straight before answering; if it means that researching will go beyond the deadline, let the reporter know, then get the information anyway. This approach is responsive without making room for the kinds of mistakes that pressure can foster.

Errors

If a story emanating from the hospital is published with a gross error, most editors will publish a retraction or correction. If the error was in copy provided by the hospital, this fact should be made very clear when asking for a correction. Insignificant errors should be ignored. Editors are concerned with libel and are often eager to set the record straight if they made an honest error. However, petty items such as misspelled names, unless the misspelling could cause serious embarrassment, should be forgotten.

An effective way of handling errors or press statements that are disagreed with is through a letter to the editor for publication. By finding something in the article that can be praised, the issue can then be expanded on, making the correction without ever referring to the error. Most editors willingly publish letters that expound on, or correct in a polite and civilized fashion, an article that has been in print. Few are eager to print or broadcast letters that call their skills or the skills of their staff into question. A reporter's or editor's integrity should never, never be questioned; this will destroy any chance of salvaging positive press relations and provide the press the opportunity to investigate the hospital in depth and detail. Members of the press, with few exceptions, take pride in their ethical standards, much the same as do professional practitioners of public relations.

Weeklies

Almost every hospital in the United States is within the circulation area of at least one daily and one or more weekly newspapers. The public relations director should prepare news that caters to the special needs of these papers, bearing in mind their deadlines and the particular orientation of these outlets. In particular, weekly newspapers tend to be people-oriented and feature-oriented; they shy away from timely or breaking news, especially when they compete with dailies. Weeklies are frequently open to stories about employees who live in their service area. By getting to know the editors and their requirements, a working partnership can be established.

Sunday editions

Large Sunday editions are compiled throughout the week, with different deadlines for special sections; making use of these sections requires knowing what these special deadlines are. Large circulation papers may have a Sunday editor responsible for those editions only.

Sunday magazine sections, usually with a special magazine editor, may be ready for press as much as a week in advance. If the magazine is sent out for printing, the deadline could be as much as four to six weeks in advance.

Guest columns

An administrator with time and talent or a good ghostwriter can exert considerable influence in the community by writing a weekly column for small community newspapers. In addition, recent public interest in wellness and related topics has created the opportunity for a hospital's health educator or a physician on staff to provide a column in this area. Both types of columns enhance the hospital's position as being responsive to and concerned about the community.

Saying thanks

Public relations practitioners who storm into an editor's office, demanding an explanation of why their latest news release was not used, are not likely to have future releases used. Practitioners who write an occasional thoughtful thank-you note to the editor for editorials, staff-written features, or evenhanded coverage of a board meeting are likely to find a receptive audience for news releases. However, thanking an editor for using a release seems, at best, unnecessary and the less said about such the better.

There are many ways of saying thank you to those in the news media, but there is only one best way to say thanks. It is worthwhile to seek out that best way and use it.

A case in point: A television news reporter, at your suggestion, covers a new unit at the hospital. The piece is sensitive, accurate, and goes a long way toward generating public understanding for and support of the hospital's efforts. How do you thank that reporter?

You could call the reporter on the phone: "Just wanted to tell you what a fine job you did on that CAT scan story. Come by any time."

You could write the reporter a letter: "Your story on the new CAT scanner at Hometown General was a top-notch piece of video journalism. On behalf of the hospital and myself, I want to thank you for your efforts."

You could write the FCC a letter: "We at Hometown General recently added a sophisticated CAT scanner to our arsenal of diagnostic equipment. However, it was not being effectively utilized as a result of serious public misunderstanding. (Insert name), a reporter with WXXX-TV, put together a sensitive, accurate piece of reporting that has gone a long way toward generating public understanding for, and support of, the hospital's efforts. Please keep this letter on file for consideration when WXXX's license comes up for renewal. cc: Station Manager, WXXX."

Which is the most effective way of saying thanks? Clearly, the last is. You are doing the station an important favor and giving the reporter the credit. The reporter will see your letter only after it has been routed from the station manager to the news director to the assignments editor. Management will have seen it first, and he will know it. The next time you call, the reporter will be a little more inclined to respond, and the bosses will be a little more inclined to approve the next story idea on your hospital. In this way, your act of common courtesy will pay dividends.

Although the idea of writing to the FCC works only with broadcasters, the idea of thanking the person in charge, be he station manager or publisher or editor-in-chief has merit. The person being thanked—the reporter—will receive credit within his organization, making the thanks pay dividends.

Releasing news to the press

For general news—promotions, awards, new personnel, new equipment, and so forth—a news release sent to the appropriate media is adequate. It provides the best opportunity to get the names, dates, and figures printed accurately and completely. With a release of this nature, the paper has the opportunity to expand, cut, or drop the story.

The news may have a timeliness requiring its release on a certain day and time, which should be indicated on the release, for example, "For release Wednesday, October 26, after 2:00 p.m." However, in most cases, the release should state "for immediate release."

Copy should be typed or clearly photocopied on hospital letterhead or special news release stationery. Carbon copies should never be sent to newspapers. Two cautions: some editors choose not to honor an embargo that requests holding a release for a specific date, and some editors are openly contemptuous of news release stationery that calls attention to itself through bright colors or gaudy artwork. Low-key letterhead will let the news carry the day.

The most effective way of distributing a news release is carrying it to editors or reporters in person, preferably letting them know in advance. In this way, if they are interested, follow-up questions can be answered immediately. The opportunity also exists to provide a lead to another article or story they might find intriguing. However, if the news is minor or if time is not available, first-class mail is appropriate. Calling to mention that the news is in the mail not only emphasizes the news, but also alerts the editors or reporters to basic topics that may intrigue them. Again, deadline times are too hectic to intrude with delivering a release or calling a reporter.

Sometimes, though, it may be necessary to phone in a story. For example, 30 minutes before deadline a member of the city council has died in the hospital. After making sure that the family has been notified, the next step is to call local city editors and give them the basic facts. From there, they can develop the story, and they will appreciate the sensitivity to their needs.

For feature stories such as the successful performance of unusual surgery, in contrast to hard news, editors may wish to send a reporter and photographer to the hospital to cover the story. The role of the public relations director is to arrange the necessary interviews, provide background materials, stage photographs, and, in particular, protect the patient's right to privacy.

In communities with competing newspapers or television stations, giving exclusive stories must be done very carefully. If a reporter is working on an exclusive and a competing reporter calls on that story, the first one should be informed that, for reasons beyond control, the story is no longer an exclusive. Although a measure of coverage may be lost, immeasurable gains in credibility will be attained.

There is public relations value in hometown news. Of course, the activities of employees are a constant source of hometown news. And other sources exist. That an out-of-town person survives a critical operation in the hospital may be of limited interest to local newspapers, but the hometown or community newspaper might consider this front-page news. However, an important step is to get clearance from the patient first.

Keeping a record of the successes and failures of press communication efforts helps in the evaluation of the public relations program and serves as a reminder for future efforts. However, like all programs and projects, each release must have its own internal justification based on its ability to promote one or more of the hospital's goals and objectives. By adhering to this principle, public relations can avoid the trap of "If this is Tuesday, it must be time for a press release."

Preparing a news release

The more professionally a news release is prepared, the better its chance of success. Reporters learn in basic journalism classes to answer the following questions: who, what, when, where, why, and how. They also learn the inverted pyramid, to put the most important news first so an editor can cut a story from the bottom without losing any vital information. In other words, news in the fourth paragraph is buried.

In good news stories, reporters lean heavily on concise quotes attributed to an authority. Following this example increases the chances of getting stories in print. Short words, short sentences, and short paragraphs should be used. As few as two sentences can form an effective paragraph in a news release. Adjectives, personal pronouns, comments, and personal opinions should be avoided, outside of attributed quotations. These limits provide a good reason for using attributed comments liberally. A good style-book will provide answers to questions about the use of figures, abbreviations, titles, and other matters of style required in effective news release copy.

The standard format for releases is on 8½-inch by 11-inch white paper, using hospital letterhead or news release stationery. The hospital's name and address, the name of the public relations contact person, with title and telephone number, should be included (a home telephone number may be included if the public relations contact is on call). Room should be left for editors to provide instructions. Catchy headlines can help, but they are often rewritten.

If the story is longer than one page, adding the word *more* in the center of the bottom of the first page is helpful. At the top of each following page, in the upper left-hand corner, a one-word or two-word slug identifies the page, for example, "Hospital Expansion." Beneath or beside this is the number of the page in newspaper style: "add one" for page two, "add two" for page three, and so forth. The end of the release is indicated with "###" or "-30-" (see examples, next four pages).

Photographs for the news media

Some stories for the news media will warrant an accompanying photograph. There may be times when all a release needs is a photo and caption. Newspapers require black-and-white glossies of at least 5 inches by 7 inches. Television requires 35-mm slides in a special format. Technical directors at local stations will provide specific dimensions if asked.

News From...

Hometown General Hospital

FOR MORE INFORMATION, CONTACT:
Mary Spokesperson, Director of Public Relations
312/555-1234
312/555-8888 (Home phone)

FOR IMMEDIATE RELEASE

SHORT-STAY SURGERY CENTER OPENED

Hometown, FL (January 9, 1984)--Hometown General Hospital will officially open its new Percy Scott Short-Stay Surgery Center today, according to William J. Ceo, hospital president. "Our new short-stay surgery center will bring an added dimension of service to residents of Hometown," Ceo stated. Many routine surgical procedures will no longer necessitate an overnight stay, which will be a real convenience for hospital patients and families.

The new center is located adjacent to the hospital, at Summit Street and Second Avenue, to provide a convenient and familiar location with ample parking. The center will be open Monday through Saturday.

Speaking on behalf of the medical staff, Charles Simpson, M.D., chief of

(more)

Surgery Center/2

PRESS RELEASE FORMAT Add one

staff, stated, "Our physicians are extremely pleased that Hometown's board of trustees took the initiative to build this short-stay surgery center. It will permit our medical staff to serve patients in the most efficient, convenient, and cost-effective manner when performing minor surgical procedures."

The dedication ceremony for the Percy Scott Short-Stay Surgery Center of Hometown General Hospital will take place at 1 p.m. today. Taking part in the ceremony will be Jonathan   ler, chairman of the hospital board of trustees; Dr. Simpson and other members of the medical staff; Marjorie Weeks, hospital auxiliary president; Hometown Mayor Donald J. Sullivan; Mrs. Percy Scott; and Mr. Ceo.

An open house for the public will be held at the new center from 1 p.m. to 5 p.m. on Sunday, January 15.

Hometown General Hospital, founded in 1973, is a 400-bed, not-for-profit community hospital serving the communities of Hometown, Yourtown, and Mytown.

A Public Service Message from...

Hometown General Hospital
Serving Greater Hometown Since 1973

FOR MORE INFORMATION, CONTACT:
Mary Spokesperson, Director of Public Relations
312/555-1234
312/555-8888 (Home phone)

FOR USE FROM: January 9 to Janury 15, 1984

30 SECONDS

FREE BLOOD PRESSURE SCREENINGS AVAILABLE

Hometown, FL (January 9, 1984)--Hometown General Hospital will conduct
free blood pressure screenings on Sunday, January 15, in conjunction with
the opening of its new Percy Scott Short-Stay Surgery Center.

The public is invited to tour the new short-stay surgery center, located
at Summit Street and Second Avenue, from 1 p.m. to 5 p.m. Members of the
hospital's medical staff and nursing department will conduct the blood
pressure screenings. Tours will be provided by members of the hospital
auxiliary. Refreshments will be served.

###

News From...

Hometown General Hospital
Serving Greater Hometown Since 1973

30 SECONDS

FOR MORE INFORMATION, CONTACT:
Mary Spokesperson, Director of Public Relations
312/555-1234
312/555-8888 (Home phone)

FOR IMMEDIATE RELEASE

NEW SURGERY CENTER OPENS

Hometown, FL (January 9, 1984)--Hometown General Hospital will officially

dedicate its new short-stay surgery center at 1 p.m. today. With the

opening of this center, patients requiring minor surgical procedures will

no longer find it necessary to spend a night in the hospital.

The public is invited to an open house to be held at the center from

1 p.m. to 5 p.m., this Sunday, January 15. The center is located at

Summit Street and Second Avenue.

###

Although the photograph or slide may be sent with a news release, the illustration must bear a caption, called a cutline, or other identification firmly affixed. The cutline should be short and specifically identify the illustration. The lower half of 8½-inch by 11-inch plain bond paper is used for copy, the upper half to affix the illustration.

Whether photographs are taken by staff or a professional photographer, there are several guidelines to follow:

● Permission. Do not photograph patients without a signed release on file. In all cases, the patient or an adult guardian must sign the release form, and the signature must be witnessed. A copy should be attached to the patient's medical record, and a copy should be in the public relations file. This includes photos taken by newspaper employees. The release should authorize a specific use for the photo, such as a news release, brochure, and so forth. The hospital attorney should review the standard release form, as laws vary from state to state.

● Staging. Do not crowd too many people into one picture; more than three persons is generally too many. Action adds interest to photos. Props can be used to dress up the picture and to graphically identify the hospital.

● Taking. Strive for interesting angles. Sufficient light and the appropriate film and camera (only a 35-mm or larger format, standard black and white film) are musts.

● Release. Be sure the caption, identifying the source and the photographer, is attached. Cardboard backing should be used for mailing.

Copy for radio and television

Copy for radio and television should be read aloud to be sure sentences and words flow easily when spoken. News time on the air is precious, so copy should be kept short and to the point. The format broadcasters use in presenting the news is different from newspaper copy, and the differences should be learned.

Orator or a similar typeface that, when typed in capital and lower-case letters, can be read easily is preferable. Copy in solid capital letters is very difficult to read, as is small type, and should be avoided. Material in broadcast copy that is for the announcer's information should be put in parentheses; for example, "Countywide measles vaccinations begin tomorrow (Thursday, May 2) for all preschool children . . ." This indicates what day tomorrow is if the copy is misplaced temporarily or not used on the release date. The same technique can be used to give pronunciation guides for difficult names: "John Phloguay (Flog'gie) became administrator at Memorial Hospital . . . ."

Usually the news director or news editor is the person responsible for on-the-air news broadcasts.

Some radio and television stations have large news staffs and can produce comprehensive news coverage of their service area. Many station newsrooms have telephone recording devices for producing actualities, which are sound bites to accompany the facts in a news story. A word of caution: although by law everyone must be informed when being recorded, the assumption should always be made that, from the moment the phone is answered, comments are being recorded and will be used on the air. The rise of so-called investigative journalism has led to the occasional abuse of recording equipment. If you act as though you are being recorded for broadcast, problems in talking to broadcast reporters won't occur.

Radio stations are often able to send reporters to events and press conferences to tape statements and interviews. Some have news cars equipped with two-way radios to pick up police, ambulance, and fire calls. When patients arrive in the hospital, these reporters are frequently on the scene, ready to ask questions. A plan should be cooperatively developed by the public relations, emergency service, and security departments to cope with the unexpected arrival of reporters on site at the hospital.

Television news operations are generally well staffed with reporters and camera crews. To obtain coverage from such a crew, the assignment editor must be given time to schedule coverage and reporters time to edit their stories for broadcast. Therefore, the events should be planned accordingly. Videotaping has cut the time formerly required by film chemistry, but many stations still require several hours to edit. However, several stations have begun live remote broadcasts at airtime. During one of these interview situations, access to a monitor and the use of an earpiece helps in hearing cues and questions from studio newscasters and facilitates being on top of the situation. You will be able to see when you are on camera, and you are less likely to be caught off guard.

Hospitals with broadcast-quality videotaping equipment have the potential to shoot video releases for use on local news. This is a new concept and is expensive; however, where competition is stiff, it may be worthwhile.

Television news interviews about events or activities of interest to the general public are often possible to arrange. It is also possible to become a local source on national stories related to hospitals or health care. This positions the hospital as a health care leader in the community. For stories that are not of national interest, interviews between the reporter and the hospital expert can be arranged at the station. Wellness topics have been especially well received in recent years.

For news interviews, the appearance of those being interviewed should not distract from the message. They should appear neat and be conservatively dressed. It is important to tell hospital personnel to avoid white clothes, as white reflection from television camera lights causes problems. A little facial powder cuts the glare of harsh lights and should be encouraged. If possible, public relations staff should accompany the interviewee to the station to provide moral support and handle any last-minute problems.

Television and radio talk shows offer important avenues of non-news communication. An analysis beforehand can determine whether the appearance is worthwhile. Will the appearance meet the hospital's communication objectives? Can the guest handle the most difficult questions likely to be asked? Is the show live or taped and, if taped, will it be edited? Is it a panel or call-in show? Will visual aids be shown? These factors can alter the chances for success.

Broadcast public service time—in effect, free air time for ads broadcast in the public interest—remains available, although it is no longer mandated by the Federal Communications Commission. More and more, stations are requiring groups such as hospitals to provide network-quality spots, especially at major market television stations. Specific requirements can be provided by the public service directors at local stations. ASHPR/AHA, on a fee-for-service basis, offers hospitals a series of broadcast-quality PSA messages under the title "To Your Health," that meets radio and television broadcast standards.

Other media outlets
Metropolitan magazines and regional business magazines have become widespread outlets for proactive communication efforts designed to help promote the institution's long-range goals. Because many of them work months in advance, they are poor substitutes for newspapers, radio, and television stations in reporting breaking news. But for the total picture, they can be quite effective and prestigious.

Business and industry, as with hospitals, often have internal and external newsletters—publications that might welcome by-lined columns on wellness, fitness, and other related matters.

chapter nine

Community relations

Community relations involves services that the hospital provides to the community, information it receives from the community, and cooperation between the hospital and the community it serves. There is a tremendous value to positive community relations, value that manifests itself in successful development programs, community-supported certificate-of-need applications, and census in inpatient and outpatient programs.

In recent years, many hospitals have gone beyond providing services to the sick and injured inside the hospital walls. Emphasis is shifting to expanding these services into the community and engaging in public health education and wellness programs. The extent of this expansion into the community depends upon the resources available to the hospital, its long-range plans for services, and the availability of competing services that meet community needs. The decision to embark on such projects will need the full endorsement of the hospital governing board. However, the decision should not be made in a vacuum; public relations implications of such moves must be considered. For example, the insinuation of an outpatient abortion clinic or a drug rehabilitation center into an established residential neighborhood can arouse such strong negative feelings that the entire hospital can suffer, even though there are strong health care and economic justifications for such moves.

The emergency department is usually the front-line contact with the community, along with any outpatient clinics, ambulatory service centers, or similar facilities. The emergency department can often make or break the hospital's reputation. Therefore, observing the function of the emergency operation and finding out if there are frequent complaints or any complaints at all about services is important. Frank explanations, well communicated, about the services, costs, and time related to the emergency department can do much to improve community opinion of the hospital.

The first step in any community relations effort should be the identification of the hospital's community, which may be subdivided or classified by different publics such as the elderly, various ethnic groups, the medically indigent, young families, and so forth. A comprehensive survey of the community will serve to identify these publics and help you to develop a needs assessment that can assist not only community relations but service development and marketing as well.

The Canadian health care system as operated in Quebec provides an excellent example of the benefit of this approach. Although health care is socialized under government control, the service mix is controlled at a very local level. As a result, community clinics provide the precise services their population mix requires: well-baby care in a community of young families, geriatric care in older neighborhoods, even clinics that are located in subway stations and that specialize in treating the minor problems otherwise keeping people home from work for the day. In the far less regulated, more competitive marketing situation in the United States, this same sensitive approach to community needs and expectations — in the provision of services and in the development of positive community relations — can pay rich dividends to the hospital.

The following examples of community service programs may provide a source of ideas that can spur your own creativity in developing programs suited to a specific community's and hospital's needs:

● Develop a speaker's bureau and put it to work in the community, speaking to area civic, church, fraternal, and other groups, and serving as a resource to local news and public service programming.

●Set up a training program for emergency drivers, those with all-terrain or four-wheel drive vehicles who would be available in a weather emergency or disaster, to provide transportation for key hospital personnel and others.

●Sponsor education programs on dieting, heart disease, diabetes, poison prevention, home safety, child care and emergency care for baby-sitters, child abuse, how to stop smoking, and so forth at the hospital. Where possible, tie these in with local voluntary health groups such as the Diabetes Association, and with special weeks, days, or months such as National Diabetes Month.

●Hold a community health fair, featuring screening and wellness information. Provision must be made to refer patients to physicians for follow-up when the screening identifies a potential health problem.

●Sponsor or support the development of neighborhood health clinics.

●Hold classes for expectant parents on childbirth and new-baby care.

●Having first gained the support of the hospital medical staff, offer free or low-cost pre-enrollment physicals for children going to school or summer camp.

●Sponsor a medical Explorer Scout program.

●Set up equipment to x-ray Halloween treats for razor blades and other hazardous objects.

●Work with community health groups to promote preschool innoculations and similar well-baby and well-child programs.

●Invite community groups to utilize hospital meeting facilities. Then publicize their involvement with the hospital.

●Arrange for short, regularly scheduled visits by a hospital official or physician on local radio or television talk shows to discuss medical research, wellness topics, or other areas of community interest.

●In cooperation with local clergy, arrange a health care Sunday, when sermons can focus on the role of clergy and faith in healing, the role that wellness and personal responsibility play in maintaining health, and so forth.

●Develop a mechanism for promptly informing area ministers of their parishioners' admissions, and develop supportive programs to assist ministers with their chaplaincy roles.

●Develop an outreach program to the lower grades of elementary schools to combat the fears young children might have about potential hospital admissions.

●Develop a pediatric preadmission kit that will diffuse fears children have about scheduled hospital admissions.

●Schedule regular children's day programs at the hospital to let young children actually see the facilities, thereby easing their fears. Promoted as an open house, this could include a party in the cafeteria or picnic on the grounds and a guided tour of selected areas of the hospital.

● Develop a regular program of preadmission tours for pediatric patients.

● Become active in and encourage other hospital managers to become active in local civic, cultural, political, and commercial groups to help tell the hospital story. Provide assistance to the speaker's bureau in scheduling presentations.

● Publish the hospital's annual report as a newspaper insert or paid full-page ad. Consider finding a sponsor for the ad or placement to diffuse criticism about inappropriate use of funds.

● Schedule regular meal meetings with local business, government, and political leaders, in small groups, to provide a forum for telling the hospital story and answering questions.

chapter ten

Hospital publications

Any letter or piece of printed material distributed by the hospital, even the way the switchboard answers the phone, all have an effect on the overall image of the institution. Therefore, the quality of publications and other communication tools should reflect the true character of the hospital. An annual report for a hospital that is having financial trouble should not look too expensive, and this advice also applies to any hospital recently involved in a rate increase or high-charge controversy. However, a poorly prepared, inexpensive-looking patient admission booklet can reflect unfavorably on the quality of care. The goal should be to make the quality level of communication tools appropriate to their purpose and audience.

One solution to a hospital's diverse printing needs may be provided by a national publishing organization that specializes in standard-format hospital publications.* However, these standard formats must closely match the hospital's needs; if they don't, the hospital must develop its own materials.

When producing publications, the first concern is locating a reliable, reputable local printer. Colleagues in the public relations field can provide recommendations. Touring the print shops of the three most-often recommended printers will help locate a quality printer who regularly handles the kinds of printing you require. The nature of your printing requirements will help you to determine what to look for and what to ask. Turnaround time, cost, and the ability of the staff to meet your needs are key factors to consider. A quality printer can provide counsel during the planning and production phases that can help in getting the most for the printing dollar, but to do this, the one right printer must be found. A case can be made, especially in smaller communities, for placing some or all of the hospital's printing business with the local newspaper. Although one can't and shouldn't try to buy favorable news coverage, visibility with the paper will certainly be heightened by using its presses — but pay your bills promptly! Waiting 45 or 60 days to pay may be good business, but is bad press relations in this situation.

*Names of these organizations are available from ASHPR.

Cost-effective printing

When analyzing costs of a publication, it is useful to think in terms of the unit cost of an item, that is, the cost per piece. Obviously, printing in small quantities raises the unit cost. Thus, if the hospital will have an ongoing need for an item, it pays in the long-run to print larger quantities. However, the lifespan of the publication must be taken into consideration. Photos or references can quickly date the publication and make it obsolete and, therefore, must be checked before establishing the print run.

A way to cut printing costs without lowering quality is the appropriate selection of illustrations: photos are often less expensive to create, but cost slightly more to print. Another saving is to give the printer sufficient time to avoid any overtime or rush charges. In addition, providing the printer with a detailed layout and complete copy at one time and avoiding alterations after the copy has been typeset will keep costs down. In other words, be satisfied with the copy and design before the printer gets it.

Some public relations specialists advocate pre-testing publications before entering into the expensive stages of production and printing. This technique is widely used in advertising, where a series of creative concepts will be put into print or broadcast advertising format and shown to representative samples of the intended audience. The procedure is expensive, but in a multimillion dollar campaign, the procedure is sound and cost-effective. This may or may not be the case in hospital publications, where total budgets may be low.

An effective method for hospitals that pretest important publications is to create a mock-up that closely resembles the final product, including design, art, and copy features. This mock-up is taken to objective members of the target audience and critically rated on its effectiveness of communication, attractiveness, and ability to achieve goals or objectives. Although not scientific, this approach may provide a means of avoiding costly mistakes. However, there are limits to this approach; after all, a mock-up isn't a finished piece, and the environment of the test is artificial, which may skew the test results.

Another approach that can avoid costly errors is recognizing that many members of key publics, including patients and employees, may read so poorly or with so little motivation that print communication efforts are wasted on them. Expensive, wordy patient information booklets, long the staple of admission kits, may prove ineffective if a substantial number of patients are drawn from groups with high illiteracy rates. This situation can challenge the creative and conscientious public relations director to find new, effective means of communicating with these publics.

Do publications, in fact, pay off for hospitals? Virtually all hospitals agree that they do, as evidenced by the millions of dollars committed annually to their production and distribution. Yet few have taken the effort to either evaluate their publications' cost-benefit ratio or attempted to rationalize their publications — coordinating their appearance, tone, and content — to avoid overlap or conflicting messages. To accomplish these two sound management objectives, a publications audit is required.

Publications audit
The first step in any successful publications audit is the collection and identification of all printed communication pieces from every department in the hospital. Finding all of these pieces, from four-color patient brochures to photocopied instruction sheets, can be a real challenge. They seem to proliferate more quickly than they can be collected.

The next step is to identify the purpose of each piece of printed material. This step can be accomplished by asking what it is the initiating departments intend to gain, and then classifying pieces by purpose.

The third step in developing a publication audit is developing a very specific identification of all target audiences. A comprehensive audience evaluation can help to refine publications, justify the elimination of publications, or spotlight the need for specific new publications. The audience evaluation should identify (1) target publics, (2) attitudes prevalent among each of those target audiences, and (3) the size of each target public, along with ways of reaching those publics. All of this material can be useful in the next step.

The fourth step, a very important step, is evaluation. For each piece and for the communication program as a whole, a rigorous evaluation should be conducted to ensure that the purpose of the piece is achieved and that the audience is reached. Another purpose of an evaluation is to hold waste and overlap to a bare minimum. This can be the most difficult part of the process, as sentiment and tradition should not stand in the way of a professional evaluation. As a result, traditional newsletters and brochures may have to be dropped because they are ineffective.

The fifth step is setting priorities. An effective publications audit will identify several important changes needed to put the publications program into a goal-oriented, cost-effective format. If the program is already intuitively right on track, the audit will confirm it. Unless the hospital can afford to change all publications at once, it will be necessary to set priorities based on existing supplies of brochures, costs of replacement, staff time and resources, and the relative obsolescence of the pieces on hand.

Having set priorities, the sixth and final step is production. Production involves three stages: development of content, cost-effective printing, and a system of distribution. Pretesting may be used in the content development stage to provide input into the quality and effectiveness of the final product. Designing the pieces to the purpose needed (for example, making a pediatric preadmission booklet into a coloring book) can help make the pieces cost-effective. Working closely with printers in the design stages can also identify production shortcuts that will save money through the life of the piece. Without an effective, planned system of distribution, even the most attractive, potentially effective brochure or newsletter will be worthless. For example, if a brochure won't fit in a standard envelope, costs have been added and the impact weakened. If people receive the pieces at the wrong time or in the wrong place, they may disregard them, no matter how important or informative they may be. Each piece should have its own tailored distribution plan.

Below are 10 factors to consider in looking at a communication program.

● Are copies of all publications available?

● Are all publications designed and produced to communicate a specific message to a specific audience for a specific purpose?

● Are the purposes of each communication piece clear? Could an outsider identify that purpose?

● Is the distribution system goal oriented? Are the publications reaching and being read by the target audiences?

● Is each publication cost-effective?

● Can the objective served by each communication tool be more effectively reached by an alternative communication tool, for example, a different brochure, a videotape, a poster, personal contact, and so forth?

● Are the beneficiaries of the communication tools involved in the development of those tools?

● Is there a relation between the cost of a given communication tool and the importance of the objective it serves?

● Do the various communication pieces present a unified, goal-oriented view of the institution that supports the marketing, planning, and other objectives of the institution?

● Are all audiences and all communication goals reached by the publications or communication program?

If the answer to 6 of these 10 questions is "no," a publications or communication audit is in order. Of course, the techniques for a publications audit can be used for any communication program.

Guidelines for developing printed material

Although print has long since ceased to be the only means of communicating with the hospital's various publics, it remains the basis for many effective communication programs. These guidelines are offered to help public relations directors move toward more effective communication in print:

● Keep copy brief, simple, easy to read, and oriented to the purpose of the piece.

● Do not overcrowd the page with print.

● Use large type for publications aimed, however peripherally, at elderly readers.

● Use harmonious typefaces.

● Use positive language, even when dealing with a negative situation.

● Use colored inks or colored paper stocks to enhance the clarity and acceptance of the publication, not just to decorate the publications.

● Avoid colored inks or colored paper stocks for photo reproduction if clarity of image is important.

● For newsletters, consider gang-printing colors — printing several months' worth of the color in a single large pressrun — then printing the weekly or monthly runs in black to save on printing costs.

● Use photos or artwork when appropriate to enhance copy, strengthen the message, and reinforce reader acceptance.

● Do not reinvent the wheel. Obtain permission to use copy and design ideas from other hospitals and other publications that don't compete with your service area.

● Always be sure that your publication meets the goals set for it and supports the goals of the department and the institution.

Other communication media

Videotapes have largely supplanted movies as the primary alternative to print. Other formats include slide presentations, filmstrips, exhibits, posters, and billboards. When carefully planned to meet specific needs, each can be effective in a comprehensive communication and public relations program.

At one time, slide presentations were considered an inexpensive alternative to films. However, with the advent of computer-programmed multiprojector shows, this assumption is no longer valid. However, one- or two-projector shows can be inexpensive and effective communication tools. Exhibits can also be either bargain-basement or high-budget productions. The same criteria used for judging print can be used for these and other communication media.

The various public relations and other professional communication associations hold periodic workshops and publish guides for the effective use of alternative media. However, unless hospital staff has developed skills in the production of these efforts, contracting out or hiring a consultant to provide guidance and professionalism to the first efforts is best.

*chapter*eleven

Public relations projects and activities

In addition to routine daily functions, special projects, events, and activities are an important part of the hospital's overall public relations and marketing communications program and can contribute much to department and hospital goals and objectives.

Cooperative projects with neighboring hospitals, particularly projects that assist the hospital industry as well as the participating hospitals, can be important components of the overall program. Working with other hospitals helps to spread the cost of the projects in terms of human resources and dollars. The joint venture also shows the public the true spirit of cooperation — a cooperation that can have important cost containment consequences — among health care institutions. National Hospital Week, which presents excellent opportunities to tell the hospital story, provides many ideas for cooperative projects by hospitals in a given area.

The following are projects and activities that can be used throughout the year, in addition to those suggested for National Hospital Week:

● To explain hospital costs, prepare and display an exhibit. Exhibits can be set up in hospital lobbies and in public-access buildings such as banks and shopping malls. Health careers, wellness, and other public-interest topics can also be featured in exhibits.

● Participate in career days at local schools, or sponsor annual health career days in the community. This can lead to the development of a health Explorer Scout unit that helps interested teens evaluate and pursue careers in health.

● Develop a series of public events that focuses attention on the role of new technology and other factors in hospital costs.

● Develop a hospitality program to assist the family members of critically ill patients (or very young patients) who need round-the-clock family attention.

● Preholiday luncheons for auxilians, volunteers, or garden clubs can be used as decorating parties to prepare the hospital for the holidays.

● Set aside an area and provide competent supervision for a baby-sitting service to be used by hospital visitors.

● Establish a system to identify and respond to patient complaints and problems. Such a system can prevent minor irritations from becoming major problems. A system of patient questionnaires, mailed to the home after discharge, can help evaluate the effectiveness of this patient complaint program.

● Work on a program to provide prompt access to administration and public relations for visitors, employees, and members of the community to reinforce the hospital's image of being open and caring.

● Develop a special program to keep members of the board informed of public relations programs and activities.

● Develop a fact sheet or other system to communicate the purposes of the items on the bill that were ordered by the physician and in other ways justify the costs reflected in the bill.

● Develop a system of checks to be sure that visitors understand visiting policy and accept the rules and restrictions as necessary.

● Develop a program that will position the hospital as cost-effective and caring. Wellness programs, properly communicated, have served admirably in this role for many hospitals.

These are only a few of the areas in which the activities of the hospital, and the effectiveness of the communication program related to these activities, will contribute to the goals of the institution. Each should be adapted to the institution's goals, community situation, and resources; as a group, they should serve primarily as a springboard for new ideas.

chaptertwelve

Marketing and advertising

In ancient Greek mythology, Venus sprang full-grown from the brow of Zeus. In the late 1970s, marketing arrived in almost as dramatic a fashion, appearing almost overnight as the latest in a long list of saviors of the hospital industry. For a while, marketing seemed to be little more than a buzzword that appeared, captured the imagination and attention of the industry and the public, then disappeared after fulfilling its purpose. However, marketing has a role and a substance that will not permit it to fade away. Why? Because the term defines a function that hospitals must perform if they are to survive and prosper. Because it works!

Changing role of marketing
In January 1982, the ASHPR board appointed a task force to explore the role and function of marketing

within the hospital. This group's study, published in September 1982, defined the current role of marketing within the hospital and projected its function into the 1990s. The task force identified five models for the interrelationship of marketing and public relations. The two most desirable models incorporated both functions within the organization and gave primacy to each in its own area of competence—public relations to control the institutional image management and serve as a communication resource to marketing, and marketing to handle service development and sales promotion. The three that were less than desirable found either public relations or marketing in a position of primacy, or found both functions incorporated into a single position—though this may be necessary at smaller institutions.

The task force also made eight specific recommendations designed to clarify the role of public relations in marketing communications efforts and to help public relations practitioners prepare themselves for the role of marketing communicators.

One important area where the interests of marketing and of public relations functions come together is advertising. Careful coordination of advertising messages and management of the hospital's image is vital to the long-term effectiveness of the hospital's public relations program.

Changing role of advertising

Advertising by hospitals was almost unheard of a decade ago. Its growing importance was not recognized by the American Hospital Association until 1977, when the AHA adopted a code of ethics for hospital advertising. This document is based on medical ethics in advertising and is honored largely in the breach.

As hospitals have become more competitive and more marketing oriented, a growing sense that "anything goes" has caught on. Two surveys conducted in the spring of 1983 confirmed the dramatic growth of advertising by hospitals and the trend both toward price-competitive and service-competitive ads and away from the more traditional "warm, fussy," image-oriented ads usually associated with hospitals and other service-oriented industries.*

With the exception of classified ads, advertising has, until recently, been the unchallenged domain of public relations. Many successful public relations directors considered advertising to be one more tool in their communication kit—no different than press releases. However, this approach is being challenged by hospital marketers who are less concerned with the hospital's image and position in the community

---

*These surveys were conducted by the author in partial fulfillment of ASHPR Fellowship.

than with the hospital's bottom line. In those hospitals, long-range image may be sacrificed in the name of short-term gain in census. Ultimately, the role of advertising in the hospital — its nature and function — will depend on which department within the hospital controls the budget and determines the messages. If a goal-oriented public relations department, concerned both with census-building today and image in the hospital's future directs advertising, it can be a useful public relations tool. If a bottom line-oriented marketing department directs advertising, the hospital might find itself sending out conflicting messages to its varied publics. This can lead to self-defeating confusion.

Types of advertising

There are many types of advertising available to hospitals. The most popular include radio, television, newspapers, magazines, direct mail, outdoor, and specialty. Kaiser's First Law of Advertising states that there is no best advertising medium. Each medium has its advantages and disadvantages, and each should be selected according to the institution's message, the audience to be reached, and the budget available for advertising.

Radio Until the mid-1950s, radio was a mass medium. However, with the advent of television, radio adapted to fill a new niche in the communication environment. At present, radio is a selective medium, capable of delivering a specific, targeted audience, usually at a moderate cost. Radio can reach teenagers with a message about a baby-sitting training class and business executives with a message about health care costs or a promotion for a new industrial medicine program.

Radio is generally purchased in blocks of 10-second, 15-second, 30-second, or 60-second messages called *spots*. These messages can be recorded, or they can be read by on-the-air personalities. Most stations willingly provide demographic information on audience reach. The most accurate of this information comes from Arbitron audience surveys — similar to the Nielson ratings used by television stations — which break down audiences by demographics and by time of day. Stations that cannot or will not provide such information should not be "purchased," as the impact of the messages will be difficult to judge.

Television Television is truly a mass medium. It can deliver large audiences, but is fairly indiscriminate. Unless everybody in the hospital's service area must be reached, television will probably have an unacceptably high cost per thousand. However, television is a prestige medium with an exceptionally high level of credibility — people tend to believe what they see on TV, even the ads. A small, carefully selected *flight* (an advertising term for a series of messages on a given station) of TV ads can lend credibility to a much larger purchase of ads in other media.

Television production costs are high, and, unlike radio, poor production cuts dramatically into audience acceptance. TV is a visual medium and an active medium. Slides on a screen are generally ineffective, as are videotapes that have a home-movie quality. Some commercial 30-second messages have cost more than $350,000 to produce. Therefore, before buying television time, the following question should be asked: How will our ads compare to big-budget, professionally produced ads? If the answer is "poorly," the decision to use television should be reconsidered.

Because of the technical, highly specialized nature of radio and television, a qualified advertising or public relations agency can help with the production and placement of ads. Stations provide qualified, bona fide agencies a 15 percent discount — the agency fee — that is not available to other clients. This fee generally constitutes the entire commission for the agency's services, although scriptwriting and production supervision will be billed separately. If the agency wants to charge a fee for ad placement, another agency should be found.

Newspapers Hospitals have been traditional users of ads in newspapers. These uses include classified personnel ads; announcements of educational programs, open houses, and similar events; and annual reports to the community. Such newspaper ads are generally effective, especially when carefully tailored to the audience. However, when hospitals communicate complex messages in newspapers to targeted audiences, the impact of these messages quickly drops.

Magazines The growth of city magazines and the increasing availability of regional, targeted editions of national magazines has opened a new avenue of communication for hospitals. Magazines, especially city magazines and regional issues of such magazines as *U.S. News & World Report,* have a substantial credibility. Readers of these magazines are often willing to invest a few moments in an issue-oriented ad that has more than a few words of copy.

However, the most cost-effective use of magazine ads for a hospital might involve placing an ad one time in a magazine, then reprinting and using it in a direct mail campaign to the entire target audience. The notice that this ad appeared in the magazine gives credibility, while the direct mail approach guarantees a reach that no magazine can give. Because magazine ads, especially the multicolor, full-page ads that serve so well in the direct mail role, are fairly expensive on both a per-ad and a cost-per-thousand basis, every effort should be made to get the most from the advertising investment.

Direct mail Direct mail is a useful public relations tool that hospitals often overlook as an advertising medium. Yet the direct mail advertising industry is a multibillion-dollar industry. Advertising agencies, especially those not geared to handle large-volume mailings, generally avoid recommending direct mail efforts. For the client, this can be unfortunate.

The benefits of direct mail include reduction of waste circulation (assuming access to a sound mailing list), timeliness, and controlled impact. Direct mail can be the most cost-effective means of advertising; however, an attractive message must be sent in a format that will invite readership, and the mailing list must be refined to reach and deliver all of those for which the piece is intended.

Outdoor Billboards, bench seats, and highway signs are all examples of outdoor advertising. Outdoor ads can be useful in helping prospective patients find the hospital, or they can help to reinforce the messages found in other ads. Agencies often overlook outdoor ads because, for the effort involved, they are not as profitable as radio or television. Clients often overlook them because outdoors is seen as beyond the mainstream of advertising media. However, well-positioned billboards that have highly visual, short messages that make a point can be very cost effective. Where else can

thousands be reached each day for a month or more for a few hundred dollars?

Specialty Specialty advertising includes any items imprinted with the hospital name or logo, or a message that is tied into an advertising campaign. As with outdoor and direct mail, specialty advertising is often overlooked by agencies as they do not make money from it.

Many individuals, from full-time professionals to persons right out of school, sell specialty advertising. In looking for a specialty ad salesperson, seek an experienced professional who can give advice on the effective use of the medium. In addition, someone who represents a local or national production house, rather than someone who orders from a standard catalog, can lower cost and improve the targeting and the production turnaround time.

Uses of advertising

Advertising, like all public relations tools, should be used to advance the hospital's goals and objectives through targeted communication. To be effective, it should be measurable, targeted to a specific audience, and coordinated with other messages and public relations programs produced by the hospital.

Hospitals choose to advertise when the message must reach a specific audience a specific number of times within a specific time frame. The message should not differ from other messages that the public relations department might put out (with the obvious exception of classified ads). In many cases, the messages are of such a nature that radio stations will use the ads as public service messages. In addition, these stations are often open to negotiating a "buy two, get one free" arrangement when the messages are clearly in the public interest. However, self-serving ads almost never receive this kind of treatment.

Advertising can be a glamorous, almost seductive venture, especially for the unwary or inexperienced. It is generally worth the effort to seek the advice and help of an experienced public relations or advertising counselor or agency to ensure that advertising messages are professionally produced and effectively placed. It is always worth the effort to set up, at the beginning, specific methods and benchmarks to enable the advertising campaign's effectiveness to be measured. Advertising is generally far more expensive, message for message, than traditional public relations communication efforts. That this expenditure is often justified is clear. However, unless the cost justification can be demonstrated, advertising should be avoided.

chapter thirteen

Disaster preparedness planning

When faced with a disaster, the hospital's ability to respond will be directly proportional to its preparation, that is, the planning done in anticipation of a disaster, in thinking of the unthinkable. If the hospital is caught unaware, it will have to take time to formulate a response. Those minutes can be critical. The time to think about how to respond to a disaster, a disaster that would affect the hospital and, therefore, the public relations director, is now.

Disaster checklist

To help in this planning, the following disaster checklist has been developed. It includes 20 items that can help public relations directors through the first few hectic minutes and hours and minimize the effects of a disaster from a public relations standpoint. During a disaster, public relations directors should:

●Keep administration aware of their location at all times. This may seem like a basic thought, but if public relations directors are away from a telephone, if their location is not known and disaster strikes, administration cannot afford to take time to search for personnel.

●Train two volunteers to assist in case of an emergency. It is important to have individuals who can be counted on to run messages, to answer phones, and to keep the public relations director as free as possible for responding to urgent matters. These persons should be trained in the operation of the public relations director's office, and they should be given passes that will let them through emergency security lines.

●Brief the administrator, chief of medical staff, or emergency department head nurse, depending on the hospital's structure, on press conference techniques. These persons may need to speak for the hospital in the event of a disaster, and, if the public relations director is away from the hospital, the full burden of a news conference will fall upon these individuals.

●Decide where to hold a press conference. If there is a disaster, the press will cover it and periodic press briefings will be necessary. If the hospital has a family center, it should be located in an entirely different area from the media center. Auditoriums or cafeterias are likely locations. Factors to consider include public address systems, access to outlet plugs for TV lights, sufficient seating, and accessibility to telephones.

●Identify and designate press telephone lines that will be near the pressroom. If phones are not available, the press will search the hospital for telephones that might be needed in responding to the disaster.

●Compile a survivors list for the chaplain's or the medical social services departments. If it is a community disaster, plan to call other hospitals and develop a master list. In developing the disaster plan, work with resource people such as the chaplain or social workers. They may be able to develop that list for you.

●Make a list of all reporters who call. The chaos of a disaster will work against remembering who called and what their questions were.

●Know in advance the boundaries of information that can be released and the disaster plan. A disaster is a bad time to go scurrying to the policy and procedure manual to find out what is to be done and what can be released. A disaster does not change a patient's right to privacy.

●Know who is supervising the nursing emergency area on each shift. When a disaster occurs, that person can be contacted directly and activities coordinated immediately. The nursing supervisors should be informed that public relations will screen the press so they know where to direct reporters and do not spend essential time dealing with the press.

● Take release-of-information forms to the emergency department or verify that some are kept there. In a disaster, reporters will want and expect to interview patients. If patients in the emergency department are up to this and do not mind talking, release forms should be obtained and then, on an individual basis, reporters allowed to come in and talk to those persons. If members of the press are provided limited access, they are not likely to try to obtain a greater degree of access.

● Have a disaster preparedness folder assembled, including all the information and materials needed in a disaster, such as this disaster checklist. Other items to include in the folder are important press telephone numbers, the telephone numbers of volunteer assistants, and a current list of supervisors per shift. The folder should be in an accessible place to be moved to the disaster response station.

● Notify the next of kin before releasing names. If in doubt, keep quiet. Any information that cannot be substantiated should not be released.

● Have some food. Disasters occupy time and energy for extended periods. Eating will help maintain that needed energy.

● Take a break and get some sleep. This may require going home. But leaving is better than running on a ragged edge. It is in such cases that mistakes are made, and mistakes can be critical in a disaster. The solution is to sleep and come back for follow-up. Once refreshed, public relations directors can respond effectively in their own best interests and in the best interests of their hospital.

● Stay in control. Reporters will do whatever they can to get the story, including screaming about deadlines, pushing for exclusive interviews, and mentioning past favors. The interests of the hospital and patients must come first. The press cannot be allowed to sweep those aside.

● Assign a photographer in advance to document the emergency. Using both color and black-and-white film is best, but if only one type can be used, color film should be chosen.

● Have volunteers or security personnel escort the press to the pressroom. These persons should be told in advance what to expect of the press. Reporters will not want to be confined to a pressroom. They will want to be where the action is, which is the emergency department. However, it is the job of public relations to keep the press from interfering with the proper and effective care of the patients.

● Prepare now for a stressful situation. A good disaster plan can help relieve some of that stress, but it cannot do it all. Stress management or crisis management courses are very valuable preparation.

● Gain the cooperation of the local police in advance of a disaster. Discussions with the police department and internal security personnel about how to respond in a disaster will facilitate proper implementation of the plan.

● Discuss the disaster preparedness plan with the press. If reporters know what to expect, they are much more likely to be cooperative than if they do not. They should know how the hospital would serve their interests and their needs in a disaster, what the restrictions are on patient information, and what the restrictions are on access to and in the hospital. Their feedback can provide valuable input and perhaps result in modification of the plan.

In addition to the above checklist, the following seven keys aid in effective disaster preparedness planning.

Inspiration Brainstorming will uncover ways to handle a disaster. Make lists of all resources that you might possibly use in a disaster situation. Get ideas from as many sources as possible, and make a detailed file of these items. When a disaster strikes, you are not going to have time to collect information.

Organization Write everything down. Make sure your plans are widely circulated, that you are familiar with them, and that persons who might have to pinch-hit for you know what to do.

Application Who carries out your plan? Who does it apply to? Is the blood bank involved? Is the chaplain involved? Are the volunteers involved? Let them know your role in the overall hospital disaster plan and your own plan for a public response to a disaster.

Delegation In a disaster, you cannot do everything. Designate and identify the persons who will work with you in a disaster. Orient them and give them periodic refresher training. Set periodic deadlines to update your plan.

Frustration Count on it. Nothing is going to go right. Many plans will be for naught, but you will be much better off having plans to go wrong than just doing it on a wing and a prayer.

Perspiration Sweat it out. There is going to be a lot of hard work, and nothing you do will materially affect the disaster itself. You just have to ride it out. But it won't last forever, even though it may seem as though it will.

Appreciation Thank the individuals who helped you out during a disaster. Do not forget them; you may need them again.

Working with security

Hospital public relations and security departments do not, on the surface, seem to have much in common. In fact, there are many similarities. Security is a management function, as is public relations. The responsibilities of security in the hospital include ensuring patient privacy, protecting the property of the facility and of those employees, patients, visitors, and others who are in the facility. And, as with public relations, security must be prepared to react to a crisis situation.

Medical and paramedical personnel at the hospital are prepared for crises. Nurses and others are trained to handle a sudden influx of accident victims or to evacuate a hospital wing in the face of a building fire. However, for both public relations and security departments, such situations place personnel into unaccustomed roles that will require split-second decisions. Both departments must plan ahead and establish a close working relationship if they hope to be ready for a crisis.

What are the problems a security department can anticipate in a crisis, and how do these relate to public relations? First, crowd control can quickly become a problem for security if the hospital is the recipient of a number of disaster victims, for example, if a school bus accident occurs. Parents, friends, the news media, and the curious can all be expected to turn out in force, and this crowd must be controlled in some way.

This becomes especially difficult when the news media are concerned. Reporters will want to interview victims, and television crews will want to videotape them. The problems arise when these actions either strip patients of their privacy or, in extreme cases, interfere with the medical staff's ability to provide needed emergency care. Such interference would almost never be intentional; however, in the crush of activity, it can happen, and it is up to the public relations and security departments to see that it doesn't.

Advance preparation for dealing with the news media, families, and the curious is absolutely vital. Such preparation cannot be done in isolation. Obviously, a cooperative disaster preparedness plan involving the public relations and security departments should be coordinated with the hospitalwide disaster preparedness plan. However, just as obviously, public relations and security may have to face a crisis, such as the hospitalization of a prominent person, that the hospital disaster plan would not deal with at all.

To handle a crisis where both departments are meeting and dealing with the public, security and public relations must develop coordinated plans. These plans should include liaison with local law enforcement agencies to ensure that proper security measures could be put into place at once to protect the individual, the other patients, and the hospital's property from the crowds that could be anticipated. This coordination can be extended, on the one hand, to other groups that might be involved in a disaster: school officials, airport security, the local fire department, major employers who might experience an industrial accident, civil defense, and others as appropriate. On the other hand, this coordination could extend to the news media to let them know what the plans are and seek their cooperation in a disaster. Each group has a legitimate role to play, and cooperation can work to avoid some of the corollary problems that might develop in a crisis.

There are many other areas that public relations and security departments can work on together to solve, for example, visitor control or handling criminal patients. Yet no area is potentially more important than developing a coordinated, effective response to a crisis.

chapterfourteen

Summary

There is an increasing recognition of the need for hospital public relations and marketing communications and of the fact that properly planned and executed public relations can pay. The benefits of understanding and support from key publics; of more effective recruiting, higher census, and successful development programs; and of a secure position in the health care field can all be attributed, in whole or in part, to effective, goal-oriented communication.

Hospitals operate under much public scrutiny. Because hospitals operate with large amounts of public funds and because they seem to have life-or-death powers, the populace seems to believe that it has a right to know what a hospital does and what a hospital plans to do in the future.

Too often, public relations serves as a communication "fire department," responding and reacting to crises, but doing little in the way of prevention. Goal-oriented, proactive communication programs can provide far more benefit to the institution than any public relations fire department could ever hope to accomplish.

To survive and prosper, hospitals must communicate, bearing in mind that communication is a two-way street. Hospitals must reach out effectively to employees, trustees, physicians, government, insurance companies, business leaders, voters, taxpayers, and members of other publics that are key to the institution's well-being.

National, regional, and state public relations programs conducted by various hospital associations can have little impact without supporting local communication programs. Surveys have established that, nationwide, people are more interested in local hospital issues than they are with the "big picture."

There are many ways to improve the professionalism and impact of a hospital public relations program. Public relations directors should:

● Put each project, and the program as a whole, on a goal-oriented, accountable status.

● Use and adapt the information in this manual to build a framework for effective communication.

● Read articles on hospital and related public relations and marketing programs in hospital trade magazines, public relations journals, and other sources. (See the bibliography at the back of this book.)

● Join and participate in general and hospital public relations groups on local, regional, and national levels.

● Apply the hospital public relations checklist audit to your hospital (see appendix B).

● Meet with other hospital public relations directors to find answers to specific questions.

● Contact the state hospital association for the names of qualified health care public relations and marketing communications consultants. ASHPR can also provide names or suggestions.

● Not hesitate to ask for help when it is needed. Call colleagues, hospital public relations directors in the community or state. And call ASHPR — skilled professionals are on staff to help.

Professionalism and quality are difficult to achieve in a vacuum. Participation in professional organizations can provide the contacts and the perspective needed to achieve the best in any public relations program. In the hospital and health care industry, ASHPR, the American Society for Hospital Public Relations, fills this need for more than 2,000 professional communicators.

appendixA

News media contact list

A. Daily morning newspaper: _____

    Name of editor: _____

    Address: _____

    Telephone: _____ Deadline: _____

    If paper is not published in same city as hospital:

    Name of nearby bureau chief: _____

    Address: _____

    Telephone: _____ Deadline: _____

B. Daily evening newspaper: _____

    Name of editor: _____

    Address: _____

    Telephone: _____ Deadline: _____

    If paper is not published in same city as hospital:

    Name of nearby bureau chief: _____

    Address: _____

    Telephone: _____ Deadline: _____

C. Weekly newspaper: _____

    Name of editor: _____

    Address: _____

    Telephone: _____ Deadline: _____

D. Television: _____

    Station: _____ News director: _____

    Address: _____

    Telephone: _____ Deadline: _____

    Station: _____ News director: _____

    Address: _____

    Telephone: _____ Deadline: _____

    Station: _____ News director: _____

    Address: _____

    Telephone: _____ Deadline: _____

E. Radio: _____

    Station: _____ News director: _____

    Address: _____

    Telephone: _____ Deadline: _____

    Station: _____ News director: _____

    Address: _____

    Telephone: _____ Deadline: _____

    Station: _____ News director: _____

    Address: _____

    Telephone: _____ Deadline: _____

    Station: _____ News director: _____

    Address: _____

    Telephone: _____ Deadline: _____

*appendix*B

Public relations checklist

		Yes	No
1. Public relations programming			
	a. Is PR accepted by administration as a recognized function of management?	☐	☐
	b. Do administration, board, and PR worker work under common definition of PR?	☐	☐
	c. Has administration, PR worker specified institution's publics and assigned them priorities?	☐	☐
	d. Have long-range PR goals been established, with annual objectives to be attained?	☐	☐
	e. Have any financial considerations been given to PR programming?	☐	☐

This checklist is reprinted with permission of the Tennessee Hospital Association.

f. Has any reporting system been established by which administration, board may be appraised of PR activity, make input? ☐ ☐

2. Visitor information

   a. Are main thoroughfares marked showing way to hospital? ☐ ☐

   b. Is entrance to emergency department clearly marked? ☐ ☐

   c. Is main entrance to institution clearly marked and, if needed, are there signs in parking areas showing way to main entrance? ☐ ☐

   d. Is there an information desk, clearly marked and continually staffed, in main lobby? ☐ ☐

   e. Are visiting rules, regulations posted and visitor's brochure available explaining all pertinent rules, regulations? ☐ ☐

   f. Are there signs in emergency department explaining rules, regulations, purpose, cost information, who to see? ☐ ☐

   g. Are all secondary entrances to institution secured on exterior, or appropriately signed directing visitors to main entrances? ☐ ☐

   h. Is there any method for visitor control such as passes, visitor register? ☐ ☐

   i. Are visitor regulations reported to public through news media? ☐ ☐

3. Patient information

   a. Does your institution have a brochure containing a brief history, how the hospital is controlled and operated, a description of services, and so forth? ☐ ☐

   b. Is there a brochure explaining patient rules, regulations, billing procedures, use of room equipment, a welcome from the administrator, and other information required by new patients? ☐ ☐

   c. Do you have a brochure available explaining hospital costs? ☐ ☐

   d. Do you have a patient questionnaire to be completed by the patient after, or upon, discharge that gives the patient the opportunity to "rate" services? ☐ ☐

e. Do you have a brochure for patients on special diets informing them they will not receive the regular menu and urging them to talk with their physician if they have any questions concerning 'whys' of the special diet? ☐ ☐

f. Do you have a brochure explaining the availability of special services such as those provided by auxilians, hospital chaplains, visiting clergy program, social service workers, and so forth? ☐ ☐

g. Does your institution have any system by which any member of the administrative team pays "courtesy" calls on patients? ☐ ☐

h. Do you provide patients explanatory material concerning common diagnostic procedures they may be scheduled to undergo, such as information about upper and lower GI series? ☐ ☐

4. Employee information

a. Does your institution have any kind of employee publication through which administration can inform employees of policy, activities of interest? ☐ ☐

b. Does your institution have any system through which employees can be regularly brought together, briefed by administration, and provided an opportunity to ask questions of administration, that is, departmental meetings followed by meeting of all department heads? ☐ ☐

c. Does your institution have any mechanism by which employees are continually informed of the purpose and function of each department? ☐ ☐

d. Does your institution provide every employee a manual setting out work benefits, fringe benefits, vacation policy, grievance procedure? ☐ ☐

e. Is each employee furnished a detailed job description that is kept current? ☐ ☐

f. Do you periodically explain the type of "fringe" benefits provided, and their cost to the institution? ☐ ☐

g. "Employee of the month," service awards, retirement recognition, and so forth? ☐ ☐

h. Does your institution generally have any mechanism by which employees may make work suggestions, provide administration with new ideas, and otherwise encourage employee thinking? ☐ ☐

i. Is there any "director of personnel" or equivalent person, aside from the immediate supervisor, from whom employees may obtain guidance, counseling concerning work relations, employee benefits, vacation policy, and so forth? ☐ ☐

j. Are all employees consistently reminded of the importance of proper decorum, dress, and work habits as important elements of the hospital "image" to patients? ☐ ☐

5. Public information

a. Does your institution have any auxiliary or volunteer worker program though which the public has the opportunity to provide direct support to your institution? ☐ ☐

b. If you have an auxiliary or other volunteer group, are there provisions for close and continuing communication with administration to ensure awareness and knowledge of institution policy, problems, and progress? ☐ ☐

c. Do you have any type of speaker's program, through which institution representatives are made available to civic groups and other organizations as guest speakers? ☐ ☐

d. Does your institution have available a series of "position statements" on contemporary health topics, that is, health care costs, emerging patterns of health care, the hospital's role in community health, and so forth? ☐ ☐

e. Has your institution established and maintained regular contact with news media representatives, particularly those responsible for the gathering and reporting of news? ☐ ☐

f. Does your institution regularly sponsor open house and tours so the public can get a firsthand view of its operation and facilities? ☐ ☐

g. Does your institution have any mechanism by which public sentiment can be made known directly to the board of trustees, such as through a public advisory board of community leaders, and are such board meetings open to the general public? ☐ ☐

h. Is all board of trustee passed or approved policy made available to the news media for public dissemination? ☐ ☐

i. Has your institution established or adopted a "code" or "guide" for the release of information concerning patients to news media and, if so, has it been distributed to all media and given to all employees who may deal with media? ☐ ☐

j. Does your institution regularly send news releases to all local media concerning improved or new facilities and services, changes in charges, visitor control policy, emergency department policy, and other topics of general interest to the community? ☐ ☐

k. Does your institution encourage news media to visit your institution for "enterprise" features, news stories? ☐ ☐

l. Does your institution participate in statewide, cooperative public information and education programs organized by your regional, state, or American Hospital Association? ☐ ☐

6. Special publics

a. Does your community know who your trustees are? ☐ ☐

b. Are trustees included in any kind of information program? ☐ ☐

c. Does the community know about the organization of your medical staff, and are they appraised of its officers and new members? ☐ ☐

d. Is medical staff included in any kind of information program? ☐ ☐

*appendix*C

In-house television news: focus on employees boosts morale
by Lew Riggs, Ed.D.,
and F. Thomas Krug

Tucson (AZ) Medical Center (TMC) is helping to boost the morale of its employees by making them television stars through the "TMC Television News." This monthly in-house videotaped program was designed to complement use of the hospital's house organ and other employee communication programs.

According to a labor relations attorney for the hospital, the television program probably also has helped to forestall unionism at the hospital, although it was not developed for that purpose. For example, when a union organizing drive hit the hospital, the program aided in smoothing out trouble spots. The attorney said, "It has been our consistent observation in union organizing campaigns at a large number of hospitals that the *key* issue is rarely wages or fringe benefits, but rather . . . the employees' feelings of insecurity or lack of communication about their jobs. It seems to us that the 'TMC

Reprinted, with permission, from the July 16, 1978, issue of *Hospitals* magazine.

Television News' is *most* effective in satisfying these subjective needs."[1]

In their study of factors that affect employee morale, including "subjective needs," Carey and his coauthors determined that hospital employees with the least amount of formal education tend to receive far less internal publicity than do more highly educated employees with higher job status. Yet, these authors say, "It appears that for workers at the lowest educational level (who also have the least job status) job satisfaction is correlated with the feeling that they are part of the 'hospital team.' For this group, an administrator must emphasize the value of their contributions to the total effort of the hospital and give them positive feedback on the quality of their individual performance. For example, an article in the hospital newsletter or magazine complimenting an individual worker or department for a spirit of cooperation or good performance, perhaps including a photo, would probably have its greatest effect on job satisfaction for workers at this education level."[2]

Tucson Medical Center's large work force includes many such employees, and, for the reasons cited by Carey and his coauthors, the hospital traditionally has concentrated on recognizing these employees. However, in recent years, the hospital's internal publications have been losing their influence. In analyzing this problem, the hospital determined that many of these employees were young people, members of the "TV generation." Therefore, the hospital decided to try to reach them through television. In addition, the hospital had reason to believe that television might appeal to other employees as well.

Tucson Medical Center's layout, which is totally horizontal, tends to isolate individuals and departments. Television can help overcome such isolation. For example, it is one thing to know that the hospital has a laundry somewhere on the grounds, but it is quite another to face the laundry's huge tumbling dryers and its personnel at work via a television screen.

Moreover, the hospital was expanding, and an expansion program always involves the potential for disrupting interpersonal relationships. The hospital believed that television could minimize this problem, because it is a medium that evokes personal involvement. It tends to give "celebrity" status and special recognition to anyone appearing on the screen.

Television also is a very credible source of information. A 1975 survey showed that television was the primary source of news for 64 percent of the U.S. population and the only source for 33 percent.[3] Along these lines, the hospital's labor relations attorney said, "Our experience would indicate that the percentage of employees receiving and understanding the communication over 'TMC Television News' would normally be *much* higher than if the same information were conveyed in written form."[1]

For these reasons, the hospital decided to use television as an employee communication program in order to provide information in a compelling way, to aid supervisors in increasing employees' involvement, and to develop cohesion throughout the hospital staff.

"Behind the scenes"/"on the air"

To achieve these objectives, some firm rules for the television program were established. First, because employees occasionally had complained that the hospital's publications were management oriented, it was required that, whenever possible, all employees appearing on the program be nonsupervisory personnel. Second, minimal scripting is used in order to capture candor and naturalness. Third, professionalism is balanced with an acceptable degree of amateurism. This approach allows viewers to be proud of the show, but, at the same time, to know that the participants are not professional performers and that they, too, can participate. Fourth, the program frequently uses employees' names and focuses on departments and personnel who usually do not receive recognition.

The "TMC Television News" follows the format of television network news programs. On-the-scene reports from throughout the hospital are coordinated by an anchorman in a newsroom. Each report runs for approximately two minutes and usually includes a segment in which an employee reporter interviews an employee news source. Personnel and departments are highlighted by moving the cameras into work areas. All of the hospital's 32 departments have been featured, and hundreds of nonsupervisory employees have participated in producing the program.

Each program also includes a 30-second or 60-second "commercial." These segments have publicized special offers in the gift shop, credit union membership drives, savings bonds, energy conservation contest, the hospital's suggestion program, art shows, blood drives, new employee benefits, and the United Fund. The commercials provide additional opportunities to involve employees in the program and to provide recognition.

Each program is produced in 16 hours — nine hours for planning and on-the-scene taping and approximately seven hours for editing and duplicating the tape. The program is produced in black-and-white on reusable videotape. Production equipment includes a portable videocassette recorder and camera, two editing machines and an editing controller, a character generator for captions that are shown on the screen, two studio cameras, and a switcher. The equipment cost $24,000 and was acquired through a foundation grant, but excellent programs can be produced at considerably less cost. In its first eight months, the "TMC Television News" was produced with much simpler equipment, but its quality was sufficient to generate employee enthusiasm and to win a MacEachern Citation (an award, sponsored by the Academy of Hospital Public Relations, to recognize excellence in hospital communication programs).

The program is a joint venture of the hospital's education and community affairs departments. The resources used in producing the program were acquired primarily for in-service education.

However, working on the television news program allows educational department personnel to experiment with techniques that they later can use in in-service educational productions.

The "TMC Television News" is displayed in an enclosed dining area in the hospital cafeteria. A self-repeating videotape player continuously presents the program for two days so that employees from all shifts have a chance to see the program. It is not unusual for an entire department to attend when one of its employees or the department itself is being highlighted. The program also is circulated on a mobile television cart to departments and units that request this service. The equipment is easy to use, so employees in these departments can view the program on breaks, at lunch, or in meetings. Approximately 65 percent of all of the hospital's employees view the program each month either in the cafeteria or in their departments.

Audience response

After several programs had been presented, a survey was conducted to determine the degree to which the objectives were being met. Of the 500 questionnaires distributed to employees, 110 (22 percent) were returned. As shown by the table, the responses to the first part of the questionnaire confirmed that television was an effective format for an employee information program. In the second part of the questionnaire, employees provided specific comments about the program; 87 percent were supportive of the program, and 13 percent were not. For example, in one nonsupportive comment, an employee said that, before the hospital should spend money on any informational program, it should improve patient care facilities and diagnostic equipment. In a supportive comment, another employee said that the program enhances employees' feelings that they and their jobs are important, no matter how far removed from direct patient care, and that the program even helps personnel in the same department to better understand each other's functions.

Summary

The "TMC Television News" is achieving its objectives. It fills a communication gap in an expanding major medical center, and it helps to instill institutional pride and to elevate employees' morale. Unlike the hospital's publications, the program is not identified with management by the employees but, instead, is considered to be a neutral, employee-oriented, informational activity that cuts through the complexity of the workplace in a uniquely arresting manner. Furthermore, the program appeals to employees at all educational levels. For these reasons, the "TMC Television News" has earned a prominent position in the communication program at the Tucson Medical Center.

References

1. Curtis, L. A. *The TMC Television News*, Report. Los Angeles: Musick, Peeler & Garrett. Attorneys at Law, Mar. 18, 1977.
2. Carey, R. G., and others. Improvement in employee morale linked to variety of agents. *Hospitals,* 50:85, Sept. 16, 1976.
3. Roper Organization, Inc. *Trends in Public Attitudes Toward Television and Other Mass Media 1959-1974.* New York City: the organization, Apr. 1975.

Employee responses to questionnaire on 'TMC Television News,' Tucson (AZ) Medical Center

Questions	Answers (Percentages of Total Responses)		
	Yes	No	No Opinion
Do you like the show?	85	4	12
Do you think the news stories are interesting?	89	4	6
Do you feel you know any more about TMC as a result of the show?	87	8	4
Do you like the idea of having TMC employees be news reporters?	81	4	14
Now and then we feature a specific department. Is that a good idea?	90	2	6
The show attempts to focus on employees and what they are doing. Do you think it is succeeding in doing that?	81	8	10
Would you like the show to continue?	86	3	10

bibliography

Bittner, John R. *MASS Communication: An Introduction: Theory and Practice of Mass Media and Society.* Englewood Cliffs, NJ: Prentice-Hall, 1977.

Bonnem, Shirley. *Audio-Visual Communications in the Health Care Field.* Fairfax, VA: National Audio-visual Association, 1981.

Canfield, Bertrum R. *Public Relations, Principles, Cases and Problems.* Sixth edition. Homewood, IL: Richard D. Irwin, 1973.

Commission on Freedom of the Press. *A Free and Responsible Press: A General Report on Mass Communications: Newspapers, Radio, Motion Pictures, Magazines and Books.* Chicago: University of Chicago, 1947.

Cooper, Philip D. *Health Care Marketing: Issues and Trends.* Germantown, MD: Aspen, 1979.

Cutlip, Scott M. *Effective Public Relations.* Fourth edition. Englewood Cliffs, NJ: Prentice-Hall, 1971.

Darrow, Richard W. *Public Relations Handbook.* Chicago: Dartnell, 1967.

Jaeger, B. Jon. *Marketing the Hospital.* Durham, NC: Duke University, 1977.

Kotler, Philip. *Marketing for Nonprofit Organizations.* Englewood Cliffs, NJ: Prentice-Hall, 1975.

Kurtz, Harold P. *Public Relations for Hospitals: A Practical Handbook.* Springfield, IL: Charles C Thomas, 1969.

Lesly, Philip, editor. *Lesly's Public Relations Handbook.* Englewood Cliffs, NJ: Prentice-Hall, 1971.

MacStravic, Robin E. *Marketing Health Care.* Germantown, MD: Aspen, 1977.

Nafziger, Ralph O. *Introduction to Mass Communications Research.* Baton Rouge, LA: Louisiana State University, 1963.

Oliphant, C. A. *Public Relations for Health Care Management.* Cleveland, TN: Hospital Publications, 1975.

Public Relations Society of America. *The New Communications Technology and Its Impact on Public Relations.* New York City: Public Relations Society of America, 1981.

Ragan, Lawrence. *The Organizational Press and Other Observations.* Chicago: Ragan, 1981.

Reilly, Robert T. *Public Relations in Action.* Englewood Cliffs, NJ: Prentice-Hall, 1981.

Steinberg, Charles S. *The Creation of Consent: Public Relations in Practice.* New York City: Hastings House, 1975.

45920040

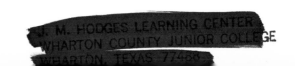

DATE DUE